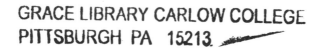

Who Will Keep the Public Healthy?

Educating Public Health Professionals for the 21st Century

Kristine Gebbie, Linda Rosenstock,
and Lyla M. Hernandez, *Editors*

Committee on Educating Public Health Professionals
for the 21st Century

Board on Health Promotion and Disease Prevention

INSTITUTE OF MEDICINE
OF THE NATIONAL ACADEMIES

THE NATIONAL ACADEMIES PRESS
Washington, D.C.
www.nap.edu

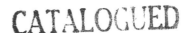

THE NATIONAL ACADEMIES PRESS • 500 Fifth Street, N.W. • Washington, DC 20001

NOTICE: The project that is the subject of this report was approved by the Governing Board of the National Research Council, whose members are drawn from the councils of the National Academy of Sciences, the National Academy of Engineering, and the Institute of Medicine. The members of the committee responsible for the report were chosen for their special competences and with regard for appropriate balance.

Support for this project was provided by Contract/Grant No. 042024 between the National Academy of Sciences and The Robert Wood Johnson Foundation. The views presented in this report are those of the Institute of Medicine Committee on Educating Public Health Professionals for the 21st Century and are not necessarily those of the funding agencies.

Library of Congress Cataloging-in-Publication Data

Who will keep the public healthy? : educating public health
professionals for the 21st Century / Kristine Gebbie, Linda Rosenstock,
and Lyla M. Hernandez, editor(s).
    p. cm.
Includes bibliographical references and index.
  ISBN 0-309-08542-X (hardcover)
  1. Public health—Study and teaching. I. Gebbie, Kristine M. II.
Rosenstock, Linda. III. Hernandez, Lyla M.
  RA440.W47 2003
  362.1'071—dc21
                          2003001043

Additional copies of this report are available from the National Academies Press, 500 Fifth Street, N.W., Lockbox 285, Washington, DC 20055; (800) 624-6242 or (202) 334-3313 (in the Washington metropolitan area); Internet, http://www.nap.edu.

For more information about the Institute of Medicine, visit the IOM home page at: **www. iom.edu.**

Printed in the United States of America.

The serpent has been a symbol of long life, healing, and knowledge among almost all cultures and religions since the beginning of recorded history. The serpent adopted as a logotype by the Institute of Medicine is a relief carving from ancient Greece, now held by the Staatliche Museen in Berlin.

"Knowing is not enough; we must apply.
Willing is not enough; we must do."
—Goethe

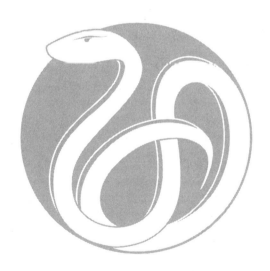

INSTITUTE OF MEDICINE
OF THE NATIONAL ACADEMIES

Shaping the Future for Health

THE NATIONAL ACADEMIES
Advisers to the Nation on Science, Engineering, and Medicine

The **National Academy of Sciences** is a private, nonprofit, self-perpetuating society of distinguished scholars engaged in scientific and engineering research, dedicated to the furtherance of science and technology and to their use for the general welfare. Upon the authority of the charter granted to it by the Congress in 1863, the Academy has a mandate that requires it to advise the federal government on scientific and technical matters. Dr. Bruce M. Alberts is president of the National Academy of Sciences.

The **National Academy of Engineering** was established in 1964, under the charter of the National Academy of Sciences, as a parallel organization of outstanding engineers. It is autonomous in its administration and in the selection of its members, sharing with the National Academy of Sciences the responsibility for advising the federal government. The National Academy of Engineering also sponsors engineering programs aimed at meeting national needs, encourages education and research, and recognizes the superior achievements of engineers. Dr. Wm. A. Wulf is president of the National Academy of Engineering.

The **Institute of Medicine** was established in 1970 by the National Academy of Sciences to secure the services of eminent members of appropriate professions in the examination of policy matters pertaining to the health of the public. The Institute acts under the responsibility given to the National Academy of Sciences by its congressional charter to be an adviser to the federal government and, upon its own initiative, to identify issues of medical care, research, and education. Dr. Harvey V. Fineberg is president of the Institute of Medicine.

The **National Research Council** was organized by the National Academy of Sciences in 1916 to associate the broad community of science and technology with the Academy's purposes of furthering knowledge and advising the federal government. Functioning in accordance with general policies determined by the Academy, the Council has become the principal operating agency of both the National Academy of Sciences and the National Academy of Engineering in providing services to the government, the public, and the scientific and engineering communities. The Council is administered jointly by both Academies and the Institute of Medicine. Dr. Bruce M. Alberts and Dr. Wm. A. Wulf are chair and vice chair, respectively, of the National Research Council.

www.national-academies.org

STAFF

LYLA M. HERNANDEZ, M.P.H., Senior Program Officer, Study Director
MAKISHA WILEY, Senior Project Assistant
MARC EHMAN, M.P.H., Research Assistant through 05/03/02
ROSE MARIE MARTINEZ, Sc.D., Director, Board on Health Promotion and Disease Prevention
RITA GASKINS, Administrative Assistant, Board on Health Promotion and Disease Prevention

REVIEWERS

This report has been reviewed in draft form by individuals chosen for their diverse perspectives and technical expertise, in accordance with procedures approved by the NRC's Report Review Committee. The purpose of this independent review is to provide candid and critical comments that will assist the institution in making its published report as sound as possible and to ensure that the report meets institutional standards for objectivity, evidence, and responsiveness to the study charge. The review comments and draft manuscript remain confidential to protect the integrity of the deliberative process. We wish to thank the following individuals for their review of this report:

Susan Addis, M.P.H., M.Ur.S., Vice-Chair, Connecticut Health Foundation, Former Connecticut Commissioner of Health

Enriqueta C. Bond, Ph.D., President, Burroughs Wellcome Fund

Patricia Flatley Brennan, R.N., Ph.D., Moehlman Bascom Professor, University of Wisconsin-Madison

Wylie Burke, M.D., Ph.D., Professor and Chair, Department of Medical History and Ethics, University of Washington

Noreen M. Clark, Ph.D., Marshall H. Becker Professor and Dean of Public Health, University of Michigan

Eugenia Eng, M.P.H., Dr.P.H., Professor, School of Public Health, University of North Carolina

Bernard Guyer, M.D., M.P.H., Chair, Department of Population and Family Health Science, Bloomberg School of Public Health, Johns Hopkins University

Jeanette Klemczak, Ph.D., R.N., Director, College of Nursing, Michigan State University

Deborah E. Powell, M.D., Dean and Assistant Vice President for Clinical Affairs, University of Minnesota School of Medicine

Joseph Telfair, Dr.P.H., M.S.W., M.P.H., Associate Professor, University of Alabama at Birmingham

Thomas W. Valente, Ph.D., Director, Master of Public Health Program, Keck School of Medicine, University of Southern California

Although the reviewers listed above have provided many constructive comments and suggestions, they were not asked to endorse the conclusions or recommendations nor did they see the final draft of the report before its release. The review of this report was overseen by M. Donald Whorton, M.D., M.P.H., WorkCare, Inc., Alameda, CA, appointed by the Institute of Medicine and Harold J. Fallon, M.D., IOM Home Secretary and Dean Emeritus, School of Medicine, University of Alabama at Birmingham, appointed by the NRC's Report Review Committee, who were responsible for making certain that an independent examination of this report was carried out in accordance with institutional procedures and that all review comments were carefully considered. Responsibility for the final content of this report rests entirely with the authoring committee and the institution.

Acknowledgments

Many people willingly shared their expertise and insights with the committee and staff during the course of this study. Their contributions invigorated committee deliberations and enhanced the quality of this report.

William L. Roper, M.D., M.P.H., conceived the idea to examine public health professional education in the 21st century, thereby prompting this study. The committee expresses its appreciation to the Robert Wood Johnson Foundation (RWJF) for sponsoring the study and, in particular, to Pamela Williams Russo, M.D., M.P.H.

Elizabeth Fee, Ph.D., commissioned to write a paper on the history of public health education in the United States, provided a tremendously thorough and extremely readable paper that elucidated for the committee the issues, events, and evolution of public health education over the past century. Additionally, her comments on an earlier draft of this report were informative and helpful in clarifying ideas. The commissioned paper by James C. Thomas, M.P.H., Ph.D., on teaching public health ethics highlighted issues of critical importance to public health education and contributed greatly to the committee's examination of the role of ethics in public health education.

The committee greatly appreciates the input of speakers whose presentations informed committee thinking including: Mohammad Akhter, M.D., M.P.H.; Elaine Auld, M.P.H.; Ronald Bialek, M.P.H.; Patricia P. Evans, M.P.H.; Virginia Kennedy, Ph.D.; Maureen Lichtveld, M.D., M.P.H.; William Livingood, Ph.D.; Samuel Shekar, M.D., M.P.H.; Harrison Spencer, M.D., M.P.H.; and Vaughn Upshaw, Ed.D., Dr.P.H. The committee extends its thanks to the Association of Schools of Public Health, the Association of State and Territorial Health Officers, the Centers for Disease Control and Prevention, the National Association of County and

City Health Officials, and the Public Health Foundation for their thoughtful and detailed input about the challenges facing public health and the educational needs of public health professionals.

The Association of Schools of Public Health was also helpful in reviewing and distributing a committee survey. Their participation was critical to the successful conduct of this survey on progress made by schools of public health in implementing recommendations of the 1988 Institute of Medicine (IOM) report, *The Future of Public Health*. The committee is grateful to the 25 schools of public health at the following universities that took the time and put forth the effort to complete the survey:

Boston University   University of Iowa
Emory University   University of Massachusetts
Harvard University   University of Medicine and
Johns Hopkins University   Dentistry of New Jersey
Ohio State University   University of Michigan
Saint Louis University   University of Minnesota
San Diego University   University of North Carolina,
Texas A&M University   Chapel Hill
Tulane University   University of Oklahoma
University of Alabama, Birmingham   University of Pittsburgh
University of Albany (SUNY)   University of South Carolina
University of California, Berkeley   University of Texas, Houston
University of California, Los Angeles   University of Washington
                                                Yale University

The work of this committee has been informed by several high quality IOM reports on relevant topics including: *The Future of Public Health* (1988); *Linking Research and Public Health Practice: A Review of CDC's Program of Centers for Research and Demonstration of Health Promotion and Disease* (1997); *America's Vital Interest in Global Health* (1997); *Promoting Health: Intervention Strategies from Social and Behavioral Research* (2000); *Health and Behavior: the Interplay of Biological, Behavioral, and Societal Influences* (2001); and *Unequal Treatment: Confronting Racial and Ethnic Disparities in Health Care* (2002). We acknowledge our indebtedness to the committees and staffs of these reports.

The committee was extremely fortunate in their staffing for this study. We wish to thank our study director, Lyla M. Hernandez, for her enormous effort in producing a clearly written, well-organized report that reflects the collective thought of the committee. Our appreciation also goes to Makisha Wiley for her administrative support, coordination of committee meetings, and maintenance of project files, and to Marc Ehman who provided research assistance throughout the initial phases of the project.

Contents

APPENDIXES

Who Will Keep
the Public Healthy?

Abstract

In a world where health threats range from AIDS and bioterrorism to an epidemic of obesity, the need for an effective public health system is as urgent as it has ever been. An effective public health system requires well-educated public health professionals. Public health professionals receive education and training in a wide range of disciplines, come from a variety of professions, work in many types of settings, and are engaged in numerous kinds of activities; however, all public health professionals share a focus on population-level health. The committee developed the following definition, used throughout the report. *A public health professional is a person educated in public health or a related discipline who is employed to improve health through a population focus.* Many institutional settings play important roles in public health professional education including schools of public health, degree granting programs in public health, medical schools, schools of nursing, other professional schools (e.g., law), and local, state and federal public health agencies. It is important that the education provided by these programs and institutions is based upon an ecological model of health. An ecological model assumes that health and well being are affected by interaction among the multiple determinants of health.

Further, it is important that public health professional education include not only the long recognized five core components of public health (i.e., epidemiology, biostatistics, environmental health, health services administration, and social and behavioral science), but that it also encompass eight critical new areas: informatics, genomics, communication, cultural competence, community-based participatory research, policy and

1

law, global health, and ethics. Understanding and being able to apply information and computer science technology to public health practice and learning (i.e., public health informatics) are necessary competencies for public health professionals in this information age in which we are vitally dependent upon data. Genomics is helping us understand the role of genetic factors in leading causes of morbidity in the United States, information that public health professionals must be familiar with to improve health. Public health professionals must be proficient in communication to interact effectively with multiple audiences. They must also be able to understand and incorporate the needs and perspectives of culturally diverse communities in public health interventions and research, and to understand and be able to influence the policies, laws, and regulations that affect health. New approaches to research that involve practitioners, researchers, and the community in joint efforts to improve health are becoming necessary as we recognize the importance of multiple determinants of health, for example, social relationships, living conditions, neighborhoods, and communities. Understanding global health issues is increasingly important as public health professionals are called upon to address problems that transcend national boundaries. Finally, public health professionals must be able to identify and address the numerous ethical issues that arise in public health practice and research.

We need high quality public health professionals contributing through practice, teaching, and research to improve health in our communities. This report provides a framework and recommendations for strengthening public health education, research, and practice skills that can be used by the institutions and organizations responsible for educating public health professionals and supporting public health education. Public health professionals' education and preparedness should be of concern to everyone, for it is well-educated public health professionals who will be able to effectively shape the programs and policies needed to improve population health during the coming century. If we want high quality public health professionals, then we must be willing to provide the support necessary to educate those professionals.

Summary

Many achievements in reducing mortality and morbidity during the past century can be traced directly to public health initiatives. The extent to which we are able to make additional improvements in the health of the public depends, in large part, upon the quality and preparedness of the public health workforce, which is, in turn, dependent upon the relevance and quality of its education and training. This report examines an essential component of the public health workforce—public health professionals.

COMMITTEE CHARGE

The charge of this committee was to develop a framework for how, over the next 5 to 10 years, education, training, and research in schools of public health could be strengthened to meet the needs of future public health professionals to improve population-level health. The committee also was asked to develop recommendations for overall improvements in public health professional education, training, research, and leadership. A wide range of institutional settings, including not only schools of public health but also degree-granting programs in public health, medical schools, schools of nursing, other professional schools (e.g., law), and local, state, and federal public health agencies, play important roles in public health education, training, research, and leadership development. This report presents conclusions and recommendations for each of these institutional settings that are directed toward improving the future of public health professional education in the United States.

DEFINITION

Public health professionals receive education and training in a wide range of disciplines, come from a variety of professions, work in many types of settings, and are engaged in numerous kinds of activities. One thing public health professionals have in common is a focus on population-level health. For purposes of this study, therefore, the committee developed the following definition: *A public health professional is a person educated in public health or a related discipline who is employed to improve health through a population focus.* Nearly all public health professionals encompassed by this definition have earned at least a baccalaureate degree.

CHALLENGES

As we begin the 21st century, public health professionals are faced with major challenges including globalization, scientific and technological advances, and demographic changes. The health of the U.S. population is increasingly affected by globalization and its accompanying environmental changes. Increased travel, trade, economic growth, and diffusion of technology have been accompanied by negative social and environmental conditions, a greater disparity between rich and poor, environmental degradation, and food security issues. There is increasing cause for concern about drug-resistant strains of emerging and re-emerging diseases (e.g., HIV/AIDS, tuberculosis, hepatitis B, malaria, cholera, diptheria, and Ebola). Along with the transmission of microbes and viruses, the increase in international trade is fostering the distribution of products associated with major health risks, for example, alcohol and tobacco.

Major challenges related to advances in science and medical technologies include important ethical, legal, and social questions. Communication technology, for example, offers increased opportunity for dissemination of health information but also requires response to the misleading or incorrect information spread through the use of this same technology. Public health informatics (i.e., the systematic application of information and computer science and technology to public health practice, research, and learning [Yasnoff et al., 2000]) offers great potential for improving our public health surveillance capacity and response but is accompanied by concerns regarding confidentiality and security of the information systems. Genomics holds the promise of helping us understand the role that genetic factors play in morbidity and mortality in the United States. However, we will need to ensure that individuals with certain genetic traits and predispositions are not discriminated against in the workplace or in obtaining insurance. While scientific advances in the biomedical field have improved the health of the public, about half of all causes of mortality in the United States are linked to social and behavioral factors and accidents (McGinnis and Foege, 1993). However, the vast majority of the nation's health research resources have been directed toward biomedical research, with comparatively few resources devoted to supporting health research on social and behavioral determinants of health (IOM, 2000).

Major demographic transformations are taking place in the United States and around the world that also present public health with new challenges. The population is aging, and this aging is accompanied by an increase in multiple chronic diseases, geriatric conditions, and mental health conditions. We are faced with the challenge of better understanding how to prevent, delay, or mitigate the effects of these diseases, thereby increasing the chances for healthful, functional aging. The U.S. population is also increasing in racial and ethnic diversity. There are large racial and ethnic health disparities reflected in increased rates among minorities of such health problems as heart disease, cancer, accidents, diabetes, and HIV infections. Improving health outcomes for all populations in American society is a major challenge for public health in the 21st century.

THE FUTURE OF PUBLIC HEALTH EDUCATION

Public health professionals have a major role to play in addressing these complex health challenges, but to do so effectively they must have a framework for action and an understanding of the ways in which what they do affects the health of individuals and populations. Several models have been proposed for understanding the forces that impact on health, that is, the determinants of health (Lalonde, 1974; Evans and Stoddart, 1994; IOM, 1999; Kaplan et al., 2000). While each model differs, determinants include broad social, economic, cultural, health, and environmental conditions; living and working conditions; social, family, and community networks; individual behavior; individual traits such as age, sex, race, and biological factors, and the biology of disease. Kaplan and colleagues (2000), Grzywacz and Fuqua (2000), and others propose that the multiple determinants of health are related and linked in many ways. A model of health that emphasizes the linkages and relationships among multiple factors (or determinants) affecting health is an *ecological model*. An example of the ecological model can be found in Figure S-1. It is important to note that the committee is not recommending any single model, but rather emphasizing the concept that there are linkages and relationships among the multiple determinants of health.

The committee believes that public health professionals must understand this ecological model. They must look beyond the biological risk factors that affect health and seek to also understand the impact on health of environmental, social, and behavioral factors. They must be aware of how these multiple factors interact in order to evaluate the effectiveness

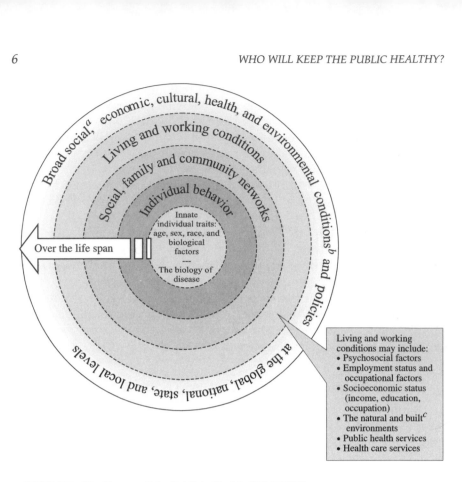

SOURCE: The Future of the Public's Health (IOM 2003).
NOTES: Adapted from Dahlgren and Whitehead, 1991. The dashed lines between levels of the model denote interaction effects between and among the various levels of health determinants (Worthman, 1999).
[a] Social conditions include, but are not limited to: economic inequality, urbanization, mobility, cultural values, attitudes and policies related to discrimination and intolerance on the basis of race, gender, and other differences.
[b] Other conditions at the national level might include major sociopolitical shifts, such as recession, war, and governmental collapse.
[c] The built environment includes transportation, water and sanitation, housing, and other dimensions of urban planning.

FIGURE S-1 A guide to thinking about the determinants of population health.

of their interventions. They must understand the theoretical underpinnings of the ecological model in order to develop research that further explicates the pathways and interrelationships of the multiple determinants of health. It is through this understanding that public health professionals will be able to more effectively address the challenges of the 21st century, including globalization, scientific and medical technologies, and demographic transformations.

While an ecological model addresses the interactions and linkages among determinants of health, an ecological *view* of health is a perspective that involves knowledge of the ecological model of determinants of health and an attempt to understand a specific problem or situation in terms of that model. Further, an ecological *approach* to health is one in which multiple strategies are developed to impact determinants of health relevant to the desired health outcomes.

The committee acknowledges that the traditional core areas of epidemiology, biostatistics, environmental health, health services administration, and social and behavioral sciences remain important for public health professional education. However, the committee believes that the following eight content areas are now and will continue to be significant to public health and public health education in programs and schools of public health for some time to come: informatics, genomics, communication, cultural competence, community-based participatory research, global health, policy and law, and public health ethics. These areas are natural outgrowths of the traditional core public health sciences as they have evolved in response to ongoing social, economic, technological, and demographic changes. For example, community-based participatory research (CBPR) can be viewed as epidemiology enriched by contemporary social and behavioral science because it incorporates what we have learned about community processes and engagement, and the complex nature of interventions with epidemiology, in order to understand how the multiple determinants of health interact to influence health in a particular community.

Education in these eight areas is important to preparing high-quality, effective public health professionals. Understanding and being able to apply information and computer science technology to public health practice and learning (i.e., public health informatics) are necessary competencies for public health professionals in this information age in which we are vitally dependent upon data. Genomics is helping us understand the role of genetic factors in leading causes of morbidity in the Unites States, information that public health professionals must be familiar with to improve health.

Public health professionals must be proficient in communication to interact effectively with multiple audiences. They must also be able to understand and incorporate the needs and perspectives of culturally diverse communities in public health interventions and research, and to inform the development of policies, laws, and regulations. New approaches to research that involve practitioners, researchers, and the community in joint efforts to improve health are becoming necessary as we recognize the importance of multiple determinants of health, for example, social relationships, living conditions, neighborhoods, and communities. Understanding global health issues is increasingly important as public health professionals are called upon to address problems that transcend national boundaries. Finally, public health professionals must be able to identify and address the numerous ethical issues that arise in public health practice and research.

Therefore, **for each of these eight emerging content areas, the committee recommends that**

- **competencies be identified;**
- **each area be included in graduate level public health education;**
- **continuing development and creation of new knowledge be pursued; and**
- **opportunity for specialization be offered.**

The committee believes that the progress made in understanding and incorporating these eight important areas into public health practice, education, and research will enable us, in the future, to identify other new and emerging areas that must be addressed. The committee also believes that it is important to enhance the development of the public health profession. While many of the things that need to be done to enhance the profession are beyond the scope of this study, certification *is* related to public health education. Within the various professions in the world of health and illness, specialty certification is common. Specialty certification attests to skills beyond the legal minimums that apply to a limited set of patients (e.g., pediatrics), conditions (e.g., infectious diseases), or interventions (e.g., anesthesia).

The range of individuals entering masters of public health (M.P.H.) programs, many with no previous health-specific education and with no access to any of the public health-related certifications currently in existence, makes M.P.H. students likely candidates for a certification program. Therefore, **the committee recommends the development of a *voluntary* certification of competence in the ecological approach to public health as a mechanism for encouraging the development of new M.P.H. graduates.**

SCHOOLS OF PUBLIC HEALTH

The basic public health degree is the master of public health (M.P.H.), while the doctor of public health (Dr.P.H.) is offered for advanced training in public health leadership. Schools of public health also offer a doctorate (Ph.D.) in various public health-related disciplines, as well as a range of masters' degrees. Schools of public health produce the bulk of degree graduates. In 1998-1999, there were 5,568 graduates from the then 29 accredited schools of public health (ASPH, 2000). Davis and Dandoy

(2001) reported that the 45 accredited programs in Community Health/ Preventive Medicine (CHPM) and in Community Health Education (CHE) graduate an additional 700 to 800 master's degree students each year. There are other programs in which students receive master's-level training in public health including programs in public administration and affairs, health administration, and community health nursing, and M.P.H. programs in schools of medicine (in 1998, 36 of the 125 accredited U.S. medical schools offered a combined M.D./M.P.H. degree).

The history of education in schools of public health has been one of evolution and change in response to new knowledge, the needs of the times, funding sources, and opportunities for improvement. Schools again are faced with the need to evolve, in part because current problems demand new knowledge and approaches, and in part because of scientific advances and the increased understanding of the determinants of health, their linkages, and their interactions. The ecological model for public health provides a focus for the discussion of future directions in public health education.

The committee determined that schools of public health have six major responsibilities. These are to:

1) educate the educators, practitioners, and researchers as well as to prepare public health leaders and managers;

2) serve as a focal point for multi-school transdisciplinary research as well as traditional public health research to improve the health of the public;

3) contribute to policy that advances the health of the public;

4) work collaboratively with other professional schools to assure quality public health content in their programs;

5) assure access to life-long learning for the public health workforce; and

6) engage actively with various communities to improve the public's health.

Education

Only a small portion of the total public health workforce receives any formal public health education, and those who do, do so primarily through certificate programs, short courses and continuing education programs, conferences, workshops, and institutes offered by a variety of institutions and organizations. While schools of public health may play crucial roles via curriculum setting, distance learning, cross-training, and continuing education for the larger public health workforce, the committee believes that the focus of education in schools of public health should be to educate masters and doctoral level students to fill many professional positions within public health, and to educate those destined for positions of senior responsibility and leadership in public health practice, research, and teaching. Some, but not all, schools of public health will continue to directly educate the broader public health workforce. **However, the committee recommends that schools embrace as a primary educational mission the preparation of individuals for positions of senior responsibility in public health practice, research, and teaching.** The committee reaffirms the importance of the long recognized core areas of public health education (biostatistics, epidemiology, environmental health, health services administration, and social and behavioral sciences). Further, the committee endorses the idea that education should be competency based and supports educational programs built upon the competency domains identified by the Council on Linkages Between Academia and Public Health Practice. However, public health professionals in the 21st century also need to understand the ecological nature of the determinants of health, that is, their linkages and relationships. Therefore, **schools of public health should emphasize the importance and centrality of the ecological approach. Further, schools have a primary role in influencing the incorporation of this ecological view of public health, as well as a population focus, into all health professional education and practice.**

The present structure of education in schools of public health is heavily oriented towards teaching the basic public health sciences, augmented by specialization in one such area. Teaching is conducted primarily by faculty with backgrounds in one of the core public health sciences with minimal participation by those in senior practice positions or those with unique skills in areas such as communication, cultural competence, leadership development, or planning. Radical change is called for and, since the goal is to inculcate a broad ecologic perspective and the amount of content material is increasingly vast, integrative teaching techniques may prove more appropriate than traditional single discipline courses. Further, the practical intention of the education would suggest that classroom teaching be substituted to the extent feasible by hands-on "rotations" with agencies and organizations of the type in which trainees are being prepared to function.

The focus on preparing individuals for leadership roles and senior practice positions requires re-design of curricula and teaching approaches to incorporate:

• enhanced participation in the educational process by those in senior practice positions or with comparable experiences, experts in medicine or its practice, or those with unique skills in areas such as communication, cultural competence, leadership development, policy, or planning;

- reconsideration of M.P.H. admission requirements to ensure that selected candidates are adequately prepared for the expanded didactic and practical training envisioned;
- vastly expanded practice rotations; and
- enhanced education for competence in specific careers (e.g., bio-statistician or health care administrator).

The committee recommends a significant expansion of *supervised* practice opportunities and sites (e.g., community-based public health programs, delivery systems, and health agencies). Such field work must be organized and supervised by faculty who have appropriate practical experience.

The range of future research in public health will also be radically different from what we see today. To a far greater degree, public health research will be transdisciplinary in nature, involving applications of basic biology and social sciences, and direct participation of the community. In the current paradigm, so-called multi-disciplinary research is the predominant research mode. Transdisciplinary research involves broadly constituted teams of researchers that work across disciplines in the development of the research questions to be addressed. Research methodology typically reflects the repertoire of the principal investigator's discipline, complemented by consultant co-investigators with additional skills. For example, at present a chronic disease epidemiologist might study the effect of an ambient air pollutant on mortality, obtaining input from an environmental chemist to help measure the independent variable (air pollutants) and a biostatistician to help explore advanced causal models.

In the future, study of the health impact of air pollutants will likely involve more broadly constituted "teams" comprised of social scientists (to measure covariation in health status caused by social factors which in the present paradigm would be viewed as "confounders"), experts in lung and cardiovascular biology (to evaluate early markers of health effect because mortality, while easily measured, is too crude an end-point given the broad and diverse population at risk), and, most novely, industrial engineers and economists to evaluate in the research context the feasibility and costs associated with alternative strategies for modifying air quality. Moreover, a far larger portion of the research portfolio is likely to be evaluative and/or intervention-focused, with interventions at the individual, community organizational, and even societal levels.

Educating individuals to conduct this research will require new approaches to the current strategy of advanced degree education at the doctorate level. The breadth of the envisioned future enterprise, and its many intersections with other scientific, biomedical and social scientific fields, suggests that an important component of science training will be directed at those who enter public health with an advanced degree in another discipline, typically an M.D. or Ph.D. Others may choose to obtain their primary doctoral-level education at a school of public health. Doctoral research candidates should have exposure to core public health disciplines as well as the eight content areas identified earlier and researchers must be trained to understand communities and to engage in transdisciplinary research. **The committee recommends that doctoral research training in public health should include an understanding of the multiple determinants of health within the ecological model.**

Research

Public health research differs from biomedical research in that its focus is on the health of groups, communities, and populations. The most striking change in public health research in the coming decades is the transition from research dominated by single disciplines or a small number to *transdisciplinary* research. Closely related to the move toward more transdisciplinary approaches to complex health issues will be the move toward more *intervention-oriented* research. The study of interventions will, in turn, dictate the third sea-change in public health research: *community participation*. Whereas the study of clinical interventions can most usually be achieved by recruitment of consenting patients or subjects, interventions at the community level require an altogether different paradigm, in which investigators and the community or population to be studied are partners. Models for such research already exist, for example the ten-year community trials funded by the National Heart, Lung and Blood Institute (Farquhar et al., 1985; Elder et al., 1986; Jacobs et al., 1986; Mittelmark et al., 1993). However, the preeminence of such research in schools of public health in the coming decades will mandate new expertise in these research modalities. In addition, such research will fundamentally alter relationships among schools of public health, the communities in which they are embedded, and the public and private agencies with responsibility for the health of these communities or populations.

The committee recommends that schools of public health reevaluate their research portfolios as plans are developed for curricular and faculty reform. To foster the envisioned transdisciplinary research, schools of public health may need to establish new relationships with other health science schools, community organizations, health agencies, and groups within their region.

Policy

Public health professionals across the disciplines of public health cannot be fully effective without an understanding of how policies are made and put into practice (Burris, 1997; Gostin et al., 1999; Gebbie and Hwang, 2000; Reutter and Williamson, 2000; Weed and Mink, 2002). An ecological understanding of public health only makes this skill set more salient; identifying social determinants of health means challenging settled practices, institutional arrangements, and beliefs that are or are not perceived to be beneficial to at least some members of the community.

Although the importance of policy in public health has long been recognized (IOM, 1998), education in policy at many schools of public health is currently minimal. Education in policy analysis, policy development, and the application of policy, must be addressed. Should schools wish to be significant players in the future of public health and health care, dwelling on the science of public health without paying appropriate attention to both politics and policy will not be enough.

Law is another essential component of education in policy. Most public health policies are embodied in or effectuated through law, and law provides the institutional framework and procedures through which policies are debated, codified, implemented, and interpreted (Burris, 1994; Gostin, 2000). From an ecological view, laws and legal practices may be important constituents of the "fundamental social causes of disease" that broadly determine population vulnerability to and immunity from illness (Link and Phelan, 1995; Sweat, 1995; Sumartojo, 2000; Burris et al., 2002); therefore a critical area in public health policy research is engagement with law.

Engagement in policy also requires a set of practical political skills, for example understanding the dynamics of community politics, identifying and working with stakeholders, identifying legal and policy structures currently influencing community health, and motivating and educating stakeholders and officials. Finally, ethics and consideration of the relationship of human rights to health play important roles in politics and policy development. They are tools through which public health professionals can interrogate their own values, formulate policy goals, and articulate a rationale for change in policy.

The committee believes that it is the responsibility of schools of public health to better prepare their graduates to understand, study, and participate in policy related activities. Therefore, **the committee recommends that schools of public health:**

- **enhance faculty involvement in policy development and implementation for relevant issues;**
- **provide increased academic recognition and reward for policy-related activities;**
- **play a leadership role in public policy discussions about the future of the U.S. health care system, including its relation to population health;**

- enhance dissemination of scientific findings and knowledge to broad audiences, including encouraging the translation of these findings into policy recommendations and implementation; and
- actively engage with other parts of the academic enterprise that participate in policy activities.

Academic Collaboration

Many senior positions in public health will continue to demand or attract physicians, nurses, trained managers, lawyers, and others (e.g., some states require that the executive of the department of health be a physician). Streamlined variations of the new practice curriculum that are oriented toward these individuals will need to be developed to inculcate the core public health competencies. Ideally, such training might be incorporated into the initial professional training experience, particularly into the curricula of medical schools and schools of nursing. The committee believes that **schools of public health should embrace the large number of programs in public-health-related fields that have developed within medical schools and schools of nursing and initiate and foster scientific and educational collaborations.**

Further, **the committee recommends that schools of public health actively seek opportunities for collaboration in education, research, and faculty development with other academic schools and departments, to increase the number of graduates in health and related disciplines who have had an introduction to public health content and interdisciplinary practice, and to foster research across disciplines.**

Access to Life-long Learning

In addition to preparing new graduates in public health, there is an existing public health workforce that requires education and training, either of workers who have no previous training in the public health aspects of their positions or of those who need to update existing skills because of evolutions in the field. While it is unclear exactly how many public health workers there are in the United States today, it is estimated that about 450,000 people are employed in salaried positions in public health, and an additional 2,850,000 volunteer their services (Center for Health Policy, 2000). Schools of public health are not necessarily primary direct providers of such training, but they do have a responsibility to *assure* that appropriate, quality education and training are available to the current and future public health workforce. The assurance role is analogous to that of the public health system, which does not always provide the necessary health services to individuals or communities but assures that their health care needs are met.

Schools can help other institutions and organizations develop training materials, and they can provide expertise in the delivery, presentation, and evaluation of materials and in the assessment of student learning. Schools are also in a good position to coordinate the sharing of "best practices" and to provide individualized education on specialized topics. Schools' broad knowledge and expertise in the public health disciplines and educational methodology positions them to assure that comprehensive, quality public health workforce education and training is available in the region served by each school. Therefore, **the committee recommends that schools of public health fulfill their responsibility for assuring access to life long learning opportunities for several disparate groups including:**

- **public health professionals;**
- **other members of the public health workforce; and**
- **other health professionals who participate in public health activities.**

Community Collaboration

Implementing effective interventions to improve the health of communities will increasingly require community understanding, involvement, and collaboration. Schools of public health have a responsibility to work with communities to educate them about what it takes to be healthy and to learn from them how to improve public health interventions. Through research and service, schools of public health have the opportunity to engage communities in the task of improving the health of the public. Community organizations and leaders have the opportunity to contribute to and influence research that has the potential to address local needs; the school can direct its expertise toward generating and analyzing appropriate local-level data and targeting significant problems. By working with the community, students in schools of public health will be exposed to far more coherent and visible community-based learning experiences.

Schools of public health will be most effective in engaging in new relationships with their communities if they take a leadership role in collaborating with other important academic units, for example, medicine, nursing, education, urban planning, and public policy. Given the premise of a future in which the boundaries of medicine and public health continue to blur, not to mention the recognition that protecting and promoting population health requires consideration of a broad array of non-biological factors, schools of public health would be well served to not go down this path alone. Therefore, **the committee recommends that schools of public health should**

- position themselves as active participants in community-based research, learning, and service;
- collaborate with other academic units (e.g., medicine, nursing, education, and urban planning) to provide transdisciplinary approaches to active community involvement to improve population health; and
- provide students with didactic and practical training in community-based public health activities, including policy development and implementation.

Further, community-based organizations should have enhanced presence in schools' advisory, planning, and teaching activities.

Faculties for Schools of Public Health

The curricular changes envisioned by the previous discussion will likely require substantial changes in the composition and backgrounds of future faculties of schools of public health, requiring both research-oriented and practice-focused components. A major barrier to increasing the emphasis on practice and service relates to faculty rewards, promotion and tenure because, within academic institutions, public health practice is not valued as highly as research activity nor is it rewarded by most academic institutions.

So that faculties with the appropriate mix of backgrounds and skills can be recruited and sustained, **the committee recommends major changes in the criteria used to hire and promote school of public health faculty. Criteria should reward experiential excellence in the classroom and the practical training of practitioners.** Unfortunately, the historical funding stream for schools of public health has fostered an emphasis on the research function. Such an imbalance has impeded maximizing the contributions of schools in practice and education. Currently, funding for schools of public health is problematic, making it difficult for schools, as well as other programs of public health education, to institute the necessary changes recommended by this report.

The committee acknowledges the major contributions of philanthropic foundations to the development of public health education in the United States and emphasizes the renewed importance of foundation support to fund new initiatives and experiments in public health education. However, greater support for public health education is needed from state and federal governments to ensure that a competent, well-educated public health workforce is available. Public health professionals, knowledgeable about the ecological approach to health and educated in a transdisciplinary fashion, are essential to preserving and improving the health of the public. Schools of public health are positioned to educate these professionals but can only do so if sufficient funding is available to develop the programs and approaches necessary to prepare future public health professionals for the challenges and opportunities of the 21st century.

OTHER PROGRAMS AND SCHOOLS

Although the primary focus of this committee's work is on schools of public health, other programs, schools, and institutions play major roles in educating public health professionals. The committee believes that to provide a coherent approach to educating public health professionals for the 21st century, it is important to examine and understand the potential contributions these other institutions and programs can make.

Graduate Programs in Public Health

A 1999 survey conducted by the Association of Teachers of Preventive Medicine (ATPM) in collaboration with the Council on Education for Public Health (CEPH) found that there were 75 M.P.H. programs in public health in the United States (Davis and Dandoy, 2001). These programs are practice oriented and are generating about one in every eight M.P.H. degrees, thereby contributing significantly to the formal educational process of public health professionals. **The committee recommends that these graduate M.P.H. programs in public health institute curricular changes that**

- **emphasize the importance and centrality of the ecological model; and**
- **address the eight critical areas of informatics, genomics, communication, cultural competence, community-based participatory research, global health, policy and law, and public health ethics.**

Medical Schools

Physicians have historically played a central, though not exclusive, role in insuring the health of the public. Beginning in the 20th century, however, the association between public health and mainstream medicine declined (although many physicians continue to lead or participate in local, state, and national public health efforts). In fact, increasing tensions resulted in a schism between medicine and public health. However, meeting the public health challenges of the 21st century will require that medical, scientific, and public health communities work together.

The committee's goal in developing recommendations for programs and approaches for public health education in medical schools is to foster improved public health training for all medical students. While such education presents challenges, there are existing examples (e.g., the programs at Duke University, the University of California at San Francisco, and the University of Southern California) that, with some modification, could produce professionals with M.D., M.P.H., and Ph.D. degrees in public health. Graduates of these programs would have the requisite training to become leaders and bridge the chasm between the two disciplines.

An ecological understanding of health and a transdisciplinary approach require physicians who are fully prepared to work with others to improve health. Therefore, **the committee strongly recommends that**

- **all medical students receive** *basic* **public health training in the population-based prevention approaches to health;**
- **serious efforts be undertaken by academic health centers to provide joint classes and clinical training in public health and medicine; and**
- **a significant proportion of medical school graduates should be** *fully* **trained in the ecological approach to public health at the M.P.H. level.**

Further, when a school of public health is not available to collaborate in teaching the ecological approach to medical students, the committee recommends that medical schools should partner with accredited programs in public health to provide for public health education.

Medical schools and schools of public health should collaborate on educational and scientific programs that address some of our most prevalent and troublesome chronic diseases, such as Alzheimer's disease, obesity, and severe/unremitting psychiatric disorders. Ongoing collaborations between schools of medicine and public health could, for example, focus on understanding how recent advances in genomics and biomedicine, in general, will have an impact on the public's health over time. Students should be exposed to dialogues between leaders in medicine and leaders in public health on central topics related to the public's health (for example, regarding the impact upon and cost to society of new-generation, subject-specific pharmaceutical products).

Therefore, **schools of medicine and schools of public health should develop an infrastructure to support research collaborations linking public health and medicine in the prevention and care of chronic diseases.**

Schools of Nursing

Nurses constitute the single largest group of professionals practicing public health. The estimated numbers available are somewhat inconsistent, given various data sources and definitions. In the 2000 estimated enumeration of the public health workforce, nearly 11 percent of the professionals identified were nurses, and there are probably a good many more practicing under more general job titles (Center for Health Policy, 2000). As is also true for physicians, all nurses at some level are a part of the public health system, given their potential contributions to the control of nosocomial infections, the identification of conditions of public health importance, and the education of patients and families about disease prevention and health promotion. Because of their important contributions, it is critical that all nurses have at least an introductory grasp of the role of public health in the community and of the principles of health promotion and disease prevention.

The roles for nurses in public health practice in public health agencies, community-based practices, and elsewhere is such that the long-standing identification of the baccalaureate degree as the entry to public health practice is likely to remain the standard, even though it is often honored in the breach. Undergraduate schools of nursing will continue to be a major source of entry-level public health workers. **The committee recommends that these undergraduate schools be encouraged to assure that curricula are designed to develop an understanding of the ecological model of health and core competencies in population-focused practice.** Because of the ongoing debate about preparation of the associate degree graduates in community skills, **the public health community should offer assistance in identifying the appropriate level and type of position for these graduates as well.** In support of sound baccalaureate-level preparation in public health nursing, **the public health community should be attentive to the need for student clinical experience, should collaborate in making appropriate sites available, and should consider ways to assure that nursing education does not occur in a vacuum apart from the full range of professionals practicing in public health.**

The graduate-level role for schools of nursing is not so clear. The inclusion of public health perspectives and skills in clinical programs in a range of specialties, as advocated by the National Organization of Nurse Practitioner Faculty (NONPF), continues the appropriate orientation of clinicians to their roles in collaboration with public health. With the exception of employment as clinicians in specific program areas, however, these are not the nurses to which public health will be looking for leadership. **Schools of nursing that offer master's degree programs in public health nursing should be encouraged to partner with schools of public health to assure that current thinking about public health is integrated into the nursing curricula content, and to facilitate development of interdisciplinary skills and capacities.**

Programs offering joint degrees in nursing and public health that bring the two schools together formally can offer a viable and effective option for advancing public health nursing practice.

Other Schools

Given the centrality of health in all our lives and the complexity of organizing collectively in a democracy to achieve it, there is a strong case to be made that curricula at all levels should include more training on health and human ecology. "Health literacy" can and should be a goal of our educational system as a whole (St. Leger, 2001). More specifically, the committee believes that the diffusion of health issues and responsibilities in society creates a need for health training in a range of jobs without health in the title. The enterprise of public health cannot succeed as a niche specialty. Creating the conditions in which Americans can be healthy requires the informed collaboration of planners, executives, and lawyers, to name just a few. There are many professions whose practitioners play an important role in health, and whose trainees are appropriate candidates for public health training.

The committee believes that public health is an essential part of training citizens, and that it is immediately pertinent to a number of professions. Specialized interdisciplinary training programs, such as the J.D./M.P.H. or M.P.H./M.U.P. (master of urban planning) can create specialists and are important. Our view, however, is that more is needed: public health literacy, entailing a recognition and basic understanding of how health is shaped by the social and physical environment, is an appropriate and worthy social goal. Further, education directed at improving health literacy at the undergraduate level could also serve to introduce persons to possible careers in public health and, in so doing, increase the cultural diversity of the future public health professional workforce. **The committee recommends that all undergraduates should have access to education in public health.**

It is beyond both our charge and our capacity to make specific recommendations about how to incorporate health into diverse curricula. Doubtless the usual challenges to curricular change will arise—faculty flexibility, scarce resources of time, and student interest. **The committee does, however, stress the importance and recommend the integration of a more accurate and ecologically oriented view of health into primary, secondary, and post-secondary education in the United States.**

PUBLIC HEALTH AGENCIES

While the committee is aware that public health professionals work in a variety of settings, there is a special relationship with the governmental public health agencies at the local, state, and federal level. These agencies have a major interest in educating and training the current public health workforce and future public health workers.

The nearly 3,000 local health departments (LHDs) in the United States vary tremendously in many ways, including size, nature of population served, economic circumstances, and governing structure. The majority of LHDs provide a wide variety of services to diverse communities with limited resources. Even with this considerable variation, more than two-thirds of local health departments provide the following core services: adult and childhood immunizations, communicable disease control, community outreach and education, epidemiology and surveillance, food safety services, restaurant inspections, and tuberculosis testing (NACCHO, 2001).

Local health departments have urgent and serious needs for upgrading the skills of those currently employed and for educating new professionals (NACCHO, 2001). Much of the training for local public health staff is obtained through the initiative of individual employees, seeking continuing education in areas of special interest or to maintain their professional credentials.

LHDs themselves provide a significant amount of direct training, primarily for narrow technical skills specific to their programs. However, LHDs can play a broader role in training and education by assessing the skills and training needs of the workforce; a role proposed in the National Public Health Performance Standards (NPHPS) (CDC, 1998), Essential Service 8 (Public Health Functions Steering Committee, 1994). Further, increased linkages between schools and programs of public health and LHDs offer many potential benefits. For example, local health department staff could serve as adjunct faculty in schools and programs of public health, thereby enhancing practical education for students. LHDs are also an important partner in community-based research because of their direct linkages to communities and awareness of local public health issues.

State public health departments are also important to the education of the public health workforce. All states, territories, and the District of Columbia have a designated entity known formally as the state public health department. The mission, authority, governance, and accountability of these public health departments vary according to the state statutes that establish them. The state health department's role in any given state is to facilitate the implementation of the Essential Public Health Services, either by carrying them out directly or indirectly through support of local public health agency efforts, and by articulating the needs of the global public health workforce to federal partners.

The responsibilities of state health departments in assuring a competent public and personal health care workforce are described in the NPHPS and include regulation, education, training, development, and assessment of health professionals to meet statewide needs for public and personal health services. States, working in partnership with the federal government are engaged in developing multiple strategies to strengthen the public health infrastructure, including the developmental and educational needs of the public health workforce.

Federal agencies' roles in public health education and research are multiple and varied including contributing to the research base that forms the content of education, testing educational approaches, helping schools develop infrastructure, supporting faculty development, and providing funding for students. Agencies involved include predecessors and current iterations of the National Institutes of Health (NIH), the Health Resources and Services Administration (HRSA), the Centers for Disease Control and Prevention (CDC), the Substance Abuse and Mental Health Services Administration (SAMHSA), and the Agency for Healthcare Research and Quality (AHRQ), all of which are branches of the Department of Health and Human Services. From the general perspective of public health education, HRSA and CDC have played the major roles.

HRSA includes the Bureau of Health Professions (BHPr), which has the stated mission to help assure access to quality health care professionals in all geographic areas and to all segments of society. BHPr puts new research findings into practice, encourages health professionals to serve individuals and communities where the need is greatest, and promotes cultural and ethnic diversity within the health professions workforce.

The programs of CDC have supported technical training for public health laboratory staff, and for program staff in tuberculosis control, sexually transmitted disease control, HIV/AIDS prevention, school health, and, more recently, in chronic disease prevention and injury prevention. The Public Health Practice Program Office (PHPPO) has provided a home base for the multi-organization Public Health Workforce Collaborative, a partnership with HRSA that involves nearly every identifiable organization representing some segment of public health workforce development. An Office of Workforce Planning and Policy was created as the organizational locus for external workforce development activities.

The potential roles for federal agencies in developing the public health workforce for the 21st century could take several forms and fall into the categories of research, development of academic programs, development of faculty, support for students, continuing education, technology development, and modeling.

Local state and federal health agencies all play critical roles in educating public health professionals for the 21st century. Local health departments are the backbone of service in public health, meeting a broad range of public health needs of the diverse communities within their areas. State health departments facilitate the implementation of the Essential Public

Health Services either by carrying out these services directly or by supporting the efforts of the local public health agencies. The importance of leadership and action at the federal level is crucial to success in educating public health professionals and the public workforce.

Therefore, **the committee recommends that local, state, and federal health agencies**

- **actively assess the public health workforce development needs in their own state or region, including the needs of both those who work in official public health agencies and those who engage in public health activities in other organizations;**
- **develop plans, in partnership with schools of public health and accredited public health programs in their region, for assuring that public health education and training needs are addressed;**
- **develop incentives to encourage continuing education and degree program learning;**
- **engage in faculty and staff exchanges and collaborations with schools of public health and accredited public health education programs; and**
- **assure that those in public health leadership and management positions within federal, state, and local public health agencies are public health professionals with M.P.H. level education or experience in the ecological approach to public health.**

While assessment of workforce education and training needs, and development and implementation of programs to meet those needs are major roles for local, state, and federal agencies, it is also important that the leaders of these agencies be fully knowledgeable and educated in public health. CDC and other public health agencies and organizations, including NACCHO, the Association of State and Territorial Health Officers (ASTHO), ASPH, and American Public Health Association (APHA), are examining the feasibility of creating a credentialing system for public health workers based on competencies linked to the Essential Public Health Services framework.

While local, state, and federal agencies all play a role in developing a competent workforce, there is a role that is primarily the responsibility of the federal agencies, that is, providing funding support for efforts throughout the system. Public health teaching, research, and infrastructure support was well funded during the 1960s and 1970s. Major decreases in funding occurred in the 1980s, and those decreased levels remained fairly constant through the 1990s. During that time, tuition and other costs continued to increase, resulting in a reduction in the amount of public health professional education actually provided.

The committee has carefully considered the rationale and feasibility of implementing recommendations to significantly enhance federal funding for both public health education and leadership development and for public health research overall, including research on population health, public health systems, and public health policy. Investment in public health education is inadequate. Federal support for non-physician graduate public health training is minimal, and funding for residencies in preventive medicine is only about $1 million (Glass, 2000).

Therefore, **the committee recommends that federal agencies provide increased funding to**

- **develop competencies and curriculum in emerging areas of practice;**
- **fund degree-oriented public health fellowship programs;**
- **provide incentives for developing academic/practice partnerships;**
- **support increased participation of public health professionals in the education and training activities of schools and programs of public health; especially, but not solely, practitioners from local and state public health agencies; and**
- **improve practice experiences for public health students through support for increased numbers and types of agencies and organizations that would serve as sites for practice rotations.***

In terms of research funding, comparatively few resources have been devoted to supporting prevention research, community-based research, transdisciplinary research, or the translation of research findings into practice. Current funding for research is focused almost entirely on two components of the ecological model of health—biologic determinants and medical cures. According to Scrimshaw and colleagues (2001), only 1 to 2 percent of the U.S. health care budget is spent on prevention and a like imbalance exists between funding for basic biomedical research and population-based prevention research. Analysis shows that at least 50 percent of mortality is due to factors other than biology or medical care (McGinnis and Foege, 1993).

Although it is not realistic at this time to propose a shift in funding for public health research to levels commensurate with the burden of need, the committee believes that significant steps in this direction are now amply justified and warranted. Accordingly, **the committee recommends that**

- **there be a significant increase in public health research support**

---

* Dr. Alan Guttmacher, because of his position as a federal employee, did not participate in discussions nor take a position regarding committee recommendations pertaining to federal funding.

(i.e., population health, primary prevention, community-based, and public health systems research), with emphasis on transdisciplinary efforts;
  • the Agency for Healthcare Research and Quality spearhead a new effort in public health systems research;
  • NIH launch a new series of faculty development awards ("K" awards) for population health and related areas; and
  • there be a redirection of current CDC extramural research to increase peer reviewed investigator-initiated awards in population health, prevention, community-based, and public health policy research, reallocating a significant portion of current categorical public health research funding to competitive extramural grants in these areas.*

Educating public health professionals to effectively respond to the new and emerging challenges requires funding support. Public health professionals can most effectively continue to contribute to improving the public's health through practice, teaching, and research *if* we are willing to provide quality support to the education of those professionals.

CONCLUSION

At no time in the history of this nation has the public health mission of promoting the public's health and safety resonated more clearly with the public and the government than now. The events of September 11, 2001, brought public health glaringly into the limelight. All citizens now have reason to understand what public health is and how the public health system interacts and shares responsibility for managing public health risks with national, regional, and local levels of government and with the health care system.

Addressing public health challenges requires an ecological approach, and the committee has developed recommendations for a framework for education, training, research, and practice based on the ecological model. The ecological model recognizes that the health of individuals and the community is determined by multiple factors and by their interactions, including biology, the social and physical environment, education, employment, and behavior (e.g., healthy ones such as exercise and unhealthy ones such as overeating).

We need high quality public health professionals contributing through practice, teaching, and research to improved health in our communities.

---

* Dr. Alan Guttmacher, because of his position as a federal employee, did not participate in discussions nor take a position regarding committee recommendations pertaining to federal funding.

This report provides a framework and recommendations for strengthening public health education, research, and practice that can be used by the institutions and organizations responsible for educating public health professionals and supporting public health education. Public health professionals' education and preparedness should be of concern to everyone, for it is well-educated public health professionals who will be able to effectively shape the programs and policies needed to improve population health during the coming century. If we want high quality public health professionals, then we must be willing to provide the support necessary to educate those professionals.

1

Introduction

The 20th century saw great achievements in public health. Vaccines and improvements in sanitation and hygiene led to reductions in mortality and morbidity associated with infectious disease. Food safety and workplace safety improved, flouridation led to improved oral health, and the decrease in motor vehicle deaths represented "the successful public health response to a great technologic advance of the 20th century" (Turnock, 2001). Indeed, the health of the U.S. population has improved dramatically during the 20th century because of public health efforts. And, without a certain level of health, people find it difficult to participate in many aspects of life, including family and community life, gainful employment, and participation in the political process. As we move into the 21st century it is important not only to celebrate the achievements of the past 100 years but also to identify and engage the new challenges to health, challenges that include globalization, scientific and technological advances, and demographic changes.

One of our most pressing tasks is to prepare public health professionals to meet these challenges. Public health has the potential to continue to improve health during the coming century, but the extent to which we are successful depends in large part upon the quality and preparedness of our workforce. As Gebbie (1999) states, "[A]t the heart of all successful public health activities—in government agencies as well as in the private and voluntary sectors—are the public health workers." To better understand what is needed to prepare public health professionals for the 21st century, the Robert Wood Johnson Foundation (RWJ) commissioned the Institute of Medicine (IOM) to *assess the past and current state of education and training (theory) for public health professionals and contrast it to future practice needs envisioned by the companion IOM study conducted by the Committee on Assuring the Health of the Public in the 21st Century. The committee's findings will be used to develop a framework for how, over the next five to ten years, education, training, and research in schools of public health can be strengthened to meet the needs of future public health professionals to improve population-level health.*

The charge further specified that the committee should deliberate the following questions:

- What is the current status of training, curricula, and research efforts at accredited schools of public health?
- How has public health education evolved over time?
- What progress has been made in responding to the recommendations of the 1988 IOM report, *The Future of Public Health*?
- What does a systematic review of the capabilities of schools of public health reveal about their capacity to educate and train public health professionals who will meet future needs for assuring population health?
- Are the broad research agendas of schools of public health consistent with future needs to assure the health of the public?
- What role can national institutions and resources play in supporting well-trained public health professionals?
- What recommendations can be made to improve public health education, training, research, and leadership?

In response, the IOM convened the Committee on Educating Public Health Professionals for the 21st Century. The committee is composed of experts in public health practice, academic public health, public health law, general graduate and continuing education, medical education, health professions training, public policy, social and behavioral sciences, occupational and environmental health, population-based and evaluation research, genomics, informatics, and communication. During the course of this one-year study the committee held five meetings (four included public information-gathering sessions); reviewed and analyzed key literature; and abstracted, analyzed, and synthesized data from catalogs and web sites of the accredited schools of public health (Appendix A). The committee also surveyed schools of public health (Appendix B) asking about progress made since publication of *The Future of Public Health* (IOM, 1988), and obtained written input from major public health organizations (Appendix C).

This report presents the committee's findings and recommendations for educating public health professionals for the 21st century. The following sections of Chapter 1 define the term "public health professional," discuss a general framework describing what public health professionals need to know and be able to accomplish, and explore how this framework guides responses to emerging public health challenges.

PUBLIC HEALTH PROFESSIONALS

Who are public health professionals? No single degree or certification characterizes this group. *Public health* has been defined in various ways. For example, Modeste (1996) defines it as

> *the science and art of preventing disease, prolonging life, and promoting health and efficiency through organized community effort for the sanitation of the environment, control of communicable infections, education in personal hygiene, organization of medical and nursing services, and the development of the social machinery to ensure everyone a standard of living, adequate for the maintenance of health.*

The Future of Public Health (IOM, 1988) defined the *mission* of public health as "fulfilling society's interest in assuring conditions in which people can be healthy." Turnock (2001), elaborating on this description, identified the activities of public health as including "organized community efforts to prevent, identify, and counter threats to the health of the public." According to the Association of Schools of Public Health (ASPH, 1999), public health encompasses a population-focused, organized effort to help individuals, groups, and communities reduce health risks, and maintain or improve health status.

Each of these definitions has in common the understanding that public health focuses on the health of populations, that is on population-level health which addresses issues pertaining to the health of large numbers of people, involves a definable population, and operates at the level of the whole person. Therefore, *a public health professional focuses on population-level health.* But which professional categories are included? Must a person have a *degree* in public health to be viewed as a public health professional? People who work as professionals in public health have received education and training in a wide range of disciplines including medicine, nursing, dentistry, social work, allied health professions, pharmacy, law, public administration, veterinary medicine, engineering, environmental sciences, biology, microbiology, and journalism. Few of these professionals have a specific public health degree. A definition that requires a public health degree would, therefore, exclude a large number of individuals who are key to improving the health of the public.

Well then, what about identifying the specific professions that engage in public health activities? As noted above, professionals who work in public health come from diverse disciplines, for example, medicine, nursing, dentistry, social work. They receive their education and training in many different academic settings. However, most professionals so educated do not work in public health, they work in a wide variety of settings. Therefore, it is not possible to define a public health professional solely on the basis of degree or training received.

What about using the organizational setting in which work is performed to identify those who are public health professionals? This criterion would include people who work for the local, state, and federal official public health agencies. Do we also include voluntary organizations? Some voluntary organizations contribute significantly to the public's health, for example, the March of Dimes and Mothers Against Drunk Driving. Other voluntary organizations do not. There are also health care delivery organizations such as hospitals and clinics to consider. Some of their work clearly involves public health activities such as providing immunizations and mounting stop-smoking campaigns. However, the primary function of health care delivery organizations is to provide medical care to individuals rather than providing programs oriented to population-level health. Organizational setting, therefore, cannot be used to define a public health professional.

After much deliberation, the committee arrived at a definition that combines the various elements discussed above; *a public health professional is a person educated in public health or a related discipline who is employed to improve health through a population focus.* Nearly all public health professionals encompassed by this definition would have earned at least a baccalaureate degree. These public health professionals contribute to improving the health of the public in numerous ways. They develop and implement programs designed to prevent the spread of infectious diseases (e.g., AIDS and tuberculosis). They conduct research aimed at determining effectiveness of health intervention programs and at translating the results of other research (e.g., basic research) to solve real-world health problems. Public health professionals work with policy makers to translate science into practical policies. They work with communities to address the wide range of community-identified public health problems. Public health professionals also are critical to assuring that the public health system is prepared to respond to immediate challenges and threats such as those faced following the terrorist attacks of September 11, 2001.

To function most effectively, public health professionals must be well educated and trained. They must have a framework for action and an understanding of the ways in which their activities affect the health of individuals and populations, and of the multiple determinants of health. The following section provides and explores such a framework.

DETERMINANTS OF HEALTH

Why are some people healthy and others not? It seems a simple question. The answers, however, are complex and have to do not only with disease and illness, but also with who we are, where we live and work, and the social and economic policies of our government, all of which play a role in determining our health. To understand how to improve health, we first must understand the determinants of health and how they interact.

Our views of health, what it is and how to measure it, have evolved over time. Until about the mid-20th century, health was measured with negative indicators, that is, in terms of mortality and disease rates. Populations with lower mortality rates were considered healthier than populations with higher mortality rates. We continue to use mortality or disease rates as broad indicators of health in a society, for example, by comparing populations according to their infant mortality rates, or their rates of heart disease, tuberculosis, or HIV/AIDS.

In the 1950s, however, efforts to redefine health were initiated. The World Health Organization (WHO) put forth a new view of health as "a state of complete physical, mental, and social well being, and not merely the absence of disease or infirmity" (WHO, 1948). The WHO definition required a much broader view of health, and concomitantly, an evolution of thinking about the determinants of health. Lalonde (1974), in a Canadian white paper, presented a framework for health that included environment, lifestyle, human biology, medical care, and health care organization as major determinants of health. The concepts and ideas presented in this white paper encouraged analysis and exploration of the importance of individual risk factors to health. Evans and Stoddart (1994) developed a more complex model. They argued that a framework for determinants of health must provide for distinctions among disease, health, functioning, and well being. Further, such a framework should consider both behavioral and biological responses to social and physical environments. A 1999 IOM report proposed a model of determinants that illustrated how individual characteristics and environmental characteristics influence health-related quality of life (symptoms, functional status, health perceptions, and opportunity). Individual characteristics were identified as biology, life course, life-style and health behavior, illness behavior, and personality and motivation; environmental characteristics were characterized as social and cultural influences, economic and political factors, physical and geographic factors, and health and social care (IOM, 1999).

Kaplan and colleagues (2000) proposed a multilevel approach to health determinants that included pathophysiological pathways, genetic/ constitutional factors, individual risk factors, social relationships, living conditions, neighborhoods and communities, institutions, and social and economic policies as the major forces having an impact on health. They argued for an approach that builds bridges between levels, rather than emphasizing one level of determinants over another.

There are numerous models that display the contextual, layered understanding of both individual and population health (Dahlgren and Whitehead, 1991; Kaplan et al., 2000). The committee finds it most useful for present purposes to embrace the concept proffered by Kaplan and colleagues, Grzywacz and Fuqua (2000), and others; that is, there are multiple determinants of health that are related and linked in many ways. A model of health that emphasizes the linkages and relationships among multiple factors (or determinants) affecting health is an ecological model. An example of the ecological model can be found in Figure 1-1. It is important to note that the committee is not recommending any single model, but rather emphasizing the concept that there are linkages and relationships among the multiple determinants of health.

An ecological model assumes that health and well being are affected by *interaction* among multiple determinants including biology, behavior, and the environment. Interaction unfolds over the life course of individuals, families, and communities, and evidence is emerging that societal-level factors are critical to understanding and improving the health of the public (IOM, 2000). For example, epidemiologic evidence demonstrates that social support improves the prognosis and survival of people with serious cardiovascular disease; social engagement and networks slow the rate of cognitive decline in aging men and women; and more socially integrated societies appear to have better overall quality of life and lower rates of mortality from all causes (IOM, 2002). Other research demonstrates that public health outcomes are associated with neighborhood cohesiveness, stability and trust, and evidence supports the view that major variations in health among countries is a result of environmental, economic, and social and behavioral factors (IOM, 1997; Beaglehole and Bonita, 1998; Kickbusch and Buse, 2001).

While an ecological model addresses the interactions and linkages among determinants of health, an ecological *view* of health is a perspective that involves knowledge of the ecological model of determinants of health and an attempt to understand a specific problem or situation in terms of that model. For example, thinking about automobile fatalities from an ecological view would include thinking about automobile design, road design, age for licensing of drivers, use of drugs (prescription and otherwise) while driving, blood alcohol levels, enforcement strategies and traffic safety education. An ecological *approach* to health is one in which multiple strategies are developed to impact determinants of health relevant to the desired health outcomes. For example, an ecological approach to the reduction of tobacco use would include alteration in physi-

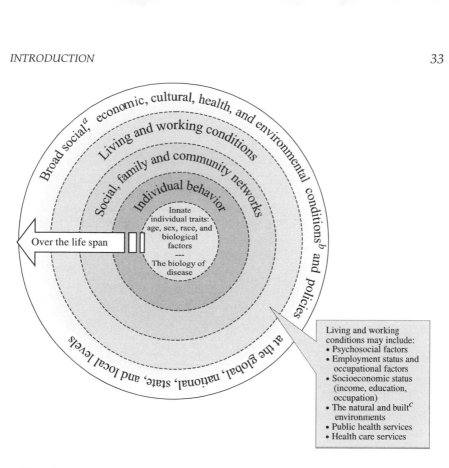

SOURCE: The Future of the Public's Health (IOM 2003).
NOTES: Adapted from Dahlgren and Whitehead, 1991. The dashed lines between
levels of the model denote interaction effects between and among the various levels
of health determinants (Worthman, 1999).
[a] Social conditions include, but are not limited to: economic inequality, urbanization,
mobility, cultural values, attitudes and policies related to discrimination and
intolerance on the basis of race, gender, and other differences.
[b] Other conditions at the national level might include major sociopolitical shifts, such
as recession, war, and governmental collapse.
[c] The built environment includes transportation, water and sanitation, housing, and
other dimensions of urban planning.

FIGURE 1-1 A guide to thinking about the determinants of population health.

cal environment (smoke-free workplaces and public places), alteration in
social environment (social marketing of tobacco prevention as a priority),
and individual behavior change (smoking cessation classes).

The committee believes that understanding the ecological model
of determinants of health is necessary to develop, implement, and
evaluate the effectiveness of interventions designed to improve health.
As McMichael and Beaglehole (2000) state,

Public-health researchers and practitioners, and those in the political and public realms with whom they interact, must take a broad view of the determinants and, indeed, the sustainability of population health. This is an ecological view of health; an awareness that shifts in the ecology of human living, in relation to both the natural and social environments, account for much of the ebb and flow of diseases over time.

Public health professionals must be aware of not only the biological risk factors affecting health; they must also understand the environmental, social, and behavioral contexts within which individuals and populations operate in order to identify factors that may hinder or promote the success of their interventions. They must be aware of the multiple factors that influence health and how those factors interact in order to evaluate the effectiveness of their interventions. They must understand the theoretical underpinnings of the ecological model in order to develop research that further explicates the pathways and interrelationships of the multiple determinants of health. With such knowledge, well-educated public health professionals will be able to design better interventions and contribute to improving the health of the public. They will also be able to more effectively address the challenges of the 21st century.

The following section explores major challenges to which public health professionals will need to respond in the coming century.

CHALLENGES

Globalization

Globalization has been defined as "the process of increasing economic, political, and social interdependence and global integration that takes place as capital, traded goods, persons, concepts, images, and values diffuse across state boundaries" (Yach and Bettcher, 1998). According to McMichael and Beaglehole (2000) globalization is "a mixed blessing for health." Increased travel, trade, economic growth, and diffusion of technology have been accompanied by negative social and environmental conditions, a greater disparity between rich and poor, environmental degradation, and food security issues. Additionally, there is cause for concern about drug resistant strains of emerging and re-emerging diseases (e.g., HIV/AIDS, tuberculosis, hepatitis B, malaria, cholera, diptheria, and Ebola).

The health of the U.S. population is increasingly affected by globalization and its accompanying environmental changes. Throughout history the movement of people and goods has impacted the health of populations. Plague was spread via trade routes, measles and smallpox traveled from Europe to America with explorers while in return the Europeans received syphilis, and the slave trade fostered the spread of hookworm and leprosy (Lee, 1999). Never before, however, has the world experienced the level of interaction that exists today. War, famine, and drought have created vast numbers of refugees; since 1990, more than 48 million people have either become refugees or been displaced within their own countries (IOM, 1997). Travel between countries has also increased. In 1996 there were more than 400 million U.S. border crossings (Barks-Ruggles, 2001). These major movements of people, coupled with the re-emergence of major infectious diseases, make it increasingly clear that the U.S. population is not immune to the threat of these emerging and re-emerging infections around the world. As the subtitle of a Barks-Ruggles (2001) article asks, "When Congo sneezes, will California get a cold?"

In addition to the movement of people, there has been a tremendous increase in the exchange of products and food, some of which is contaminated. Kickbusch and Buse (2001) reported on a cholera outbreak in Latin America that was traced to contaminated water from the ballast tanks of a Chinese trade vessel. The water, dumped in Peruvian waters, was contaminated with *Vibrio Cholerae* which infected the local seafood. Within weeks there were reports of a cholera outbreak in Peru and by the end of the epidemic almost 10,000 people across Latin America had died. As this example illustrates, diseases can be carried, not only by humans, but also by other mediums including water, plants, animals, food, and soil. In 1998 422,000 cargo-bearing aircraft underwent inspection after landing in the United States (Barks-Ruggles, 2001).

Along with the transmission of microbes and viruses, the increase in international trade is fostering the distribution of products associated with major health risks, for example, alcohol and tobacco. It is estimated that the fourth major cause of disability worldwide is alcohol. By 2025 annual tobacco-related deaths are expected to be about 10 million and the majority of these deaths will be in developing regions (IOM, 1997).

Public health professionals have a major role to play in addressing the health effects of globalization, but to do so effectively they must have sufficient knowledge and understanding to intervene in a manner that will produce improved health outcomes. This requires an understanding of the ecological model of health and of the linkages and interactions among the determinants of health. With such knowledge public health professionals will be able to develop programs and policies that maximize health outcomes in the complex environment of globalization.

Scientific and Medical Technology

Advances in science and medical technology have made major contributions to improved health. During the 20th century antibiotics and vaccines, along with improved sanitation and hygiene, led to a dramatic reduction in deaths from pneumonia, tuberculosis (TB), diarrhea and enteritis, smallpox, poliomyelitis, typhoid, cholera, and rabies. Today, however, misuse of antibiotics has resulted in emergence of drug-resistant bacteria. According to Turnock (2001):

> *the emergence of drug-resistant strains has reduced the effectiveness of treatment for several common infections, including tuberculosis, gonorrhea, pneumococcal infections, and hospital-acquired staphylococcal and enterococcal infections.*

During the last decade of the 20th century, major scientific and technological advances were made in human genetics. The Human Genome Project officially began in 1990 (Collins, 1999). By the fall of 1998, technological improvements and rapid progress led project leaders to promise the complete DNA sequence of the human genome by 2003 (Fink and Collins, 2000). Current achievements include identifying more than 10,000 genes and developing, for use in medical practice, more than 600 tests that will identify gene variants associated with diseases (Khoury et al., 2000). Further advances in genomics may identify the cause of many diseases, thereby allowing us to better understand how to prevent those diseases and promote health. Collins and McKusick (2001) predict that by 2020, gene-based "designer drugs" will be marketed for many conditions.

These major advances are accompanied by important ethical, legal and social questions. For example, if advances in genetics allow us to identify genes that are responsible for particular diseases, how will we ensure that individuals with those genetic traits are not discriminated against in the workplace or when trying to obtain insurance? Clayton (2000) writes:

> *legislators to date have said almost nothing about how and when tests for mutations that predispose individuals to develop diseases that become symptomatic only after infancy should be incorporated into clinical and public health practice. They have, however, become quite concerned that information about genetic risk factors will be used to interfere with individuals' access to employment and health insurance.*

Burris and colleagues (2000), writing about public health surveillance of genetic information, state that to be ethical, these surveillance data must be protected, and promote the health of the population, and their collection must be acceptable to the population. Suggested safeguards include: informed consent, protection of individual autonomy, confidentiality of testing results, limitation of workplace and insurance company testing, and education of both health practitioners and the general public (Khoury et al., 1999).

Ensuring that the benefits of advances in genetics are shared globally is a major challenge. Pang (2002) writes that, "the relatively rich product pipeline of genomics-based drugs will mean a tremendous increase in the demand for clinical trial sites, many of which will be in the developing countries." This raises ethical questions relating to informed consent, standard of care, and continuing availability of the drug being tested after completion of the trial.

Communication and information technologies are other areas in which major advances have occurred. Growing numbers of people have access to the Internet, providing for rapid exchange of information. Such exchange has the potential to improve population health, for example, through the spread of accurate health information. However, there is also the potential for dissemination of misleading or incorrect health information that would have a negative impact on the public's health. When used properly, however

> information technology provides tools that facilitate linking of information about the health of the public with data specific to the care of an individual patient as well as provides clinicians and patients with access to the knowledge that they need to ensure optimum health outcomes (Brennan and Friede, 2001).

Further, public health informatics (i.e., the systematic application of information, computer science, and technology to public health practice, research, and learning [Yasnoff et al., 2000]) provides an opportunity for the automation of common tasks (such as real time physician alerts on emerging disease trends detected by surveillance systems) and for improved communication among the many components of the health care and public health systems. One of the challenges of these new communication and information technologies relates to the confidentiality and security of the systems. As stated by Yasnoff et al. (2000), "[I]nformation systems are correctly perceived by the public to be a double-edged sword." As with advances in genetics, a balance needs to be achieved between individual privacy and the public good.

While scientific advances in the biomedical field have greatly improved the health of the public, McGinnis and Foege (1993) report that about half of all causes of mortality in the United States are linked to social and behavioral factors and accidents. For example, the leading cause of mortality in early to middle adulthood is unintentional injuries, the majority of which are due to motor vehicle accidents; the links between modifiable risk factors (e.g., obesity, hypertension, diet, smoking, and sun exposure) and heart disease, stroke, and cancer have been well demonstrated (Emmons, 2000).

Several studies have shown the relationship between unintentional injuries and certain risk factors, for example, accessibility to firearms, use of alcohol and tobacco, and use of seat belts (Turnock, 2001). Other research has shown the influence of psychological risk factors on disease; for example the management of diabetes is influenced by coping skills and family stresses; other research demonstrates that acute stress may trigger myocardial ischemia (IOM, 2001a).

Despite the many achievements of research, much remains to be accomplished. The vast majority of the nation's health research resources have been directed toward biomedical research endeavors that cannot, by themselves, address the most significant challenges to improving the public's health; comparatively few resources have been devoted to supporting health research on social and behavioral determinants of health (IOM, 2000). Scrimshaw et al. (2001) point out that only 1 percent to 2 percent of the U.S. health care budget is spent on prevention and that a like imbalance exists between funding for basic biomedical research and population-based prevention research. Without also addressing the social and behavioral determinants of health we are missing some of the most significant opportunities for improving the public's health.

Demographic Transformations

Major demographic changes are taking place in the United States. The median age of the U.S. population is now 35.3 years, the highest level ever recorded. By 2030 it is estimated that about 20 percent of the population (or 69 million people) will be over age 65, compared with 13 percent today, and the most rapidly growing group of older persons is aged 85 and older (Day, 1996). Population aging has been accompanied by longer lifetime exposure to potential toxic agents (e.g., tobacco and high fat food), lack of exercise that can lead to osteoporosis, sarcopenia (muscle thinning), and inadequate cardiac conditioning (Butler, 1997). The elderly tend to suffer from multiple chronic diseases, geriatric conditions, and mental health conditions such as depression and cognitive decline (Blazer, 2000). A major challenge before us is to better understand how to prevent, delay or mitigate the effects of these diseases, thereby increasing the chances for healthful, functional aging. As Koplan and Fleming (2000) put it "[I]n addition to achieving a longer lifespan for the rapidly growing aging population, increasing their healthspan must be a priority."

Another major demographic change occurring in the United States is increasing racial and ethnic diversity. White non-Hispanic people make up about 73 percent of the U.S. population but by the year 2020 the U.S. Census Bureau projects that the proportion will drop to around 64 percent because minority ethnic and racial populations are growing at a faster rate (Day, 1996). By 2050 it is expected that the Hispanic population will reach 81 million, the African American population will reach 62 million, and the Asian and Pacific Islander group will reach 41 million (Brownson and Kreuter, 1997).

Cultural diversity enriches the United States, but it also presents major challenges. Large racial and ethnic health disparities exist and are reflected in increased rates among minorities of heart disease, cancer, accidents, diabetes, HIV infections, chronic liver disease and cirrhosis, chronic nephritis, and homicide (Turnock, 2001). Access to health care and treatment is uneven:

- Twenty percent of African Americans and 30 percent of Hispanics lack a usual source of health care compared with less than 16 percent of whites; and
- minorities are less likely to receive medical treatments such as by-pass surgery, mammogram and follow-up diagnostic testing for breast cancer, antiretroviral therapy for HIV infection, and routine medication to prevent asthma-related hospitalizations (U.S. DHHS, 2002a).

Improvements in health have yet to be felt equally by all populations in U.S. society. Improving health outcomes for all components of American society, closing the gaps in access to health care, and assuring equality in quality of care are major challenges for the 21st century.

SUMMARY

The effects of globalization, scientific and technological advances, and demographic changes are profound. Yet the extent to which these effects are salutary or detrimental to the public's health depends on our responses to many changing variables. Responses that advance the health of the people of the United States and of the world depend on many factors that are beyond the purview of this report. However, public health professionals can be a formidable force for the development of positive outcomes.

The committee believes that well-educated public health professionals have an ecological view of the determinants of health. These professionals will help shape programs and policies that address the myriad health issues associated with globalization. They will be able to design and conduct research that contributes to a better understanding of the social and behavioral determinants of health, to develop culturally sensitive programs aimed at reducing racial and ethnic disparities in health, and to contribute to the debate on the ethical use and dissemination of new technologies.

The beginning of the 21st century brings new public health opportunities and challenges. This first chapter has defined public health professionals, discussed an ecological view of health and its determinants, and described challenges that face public health as we move into the 21st century. Chapter 2 reviews the history and current status of public health education in the United States. In Chapter 3 the future of public health education is explored. Chapter 4 describes the role of schools of public health in that future. The contributions to public health education of other schools and programs are described in Chapter 5, while Chapter 6 addresses the role of public health agencies in educating public health professionals. Chapter 7 is the conclusion to this report.

2

History and Current Status of Public Health Education in the United States

HISTORY

This section discusses two broad phases of public health education in America.[1] The first phase, during which independent schools of public health were first created, occurred between roughly 1914 and 1939 and was privately funded by philanthropies. The second phase, which over-lapped slightly with the first, was marked by federal and state funding, and encompasses the years 1935 to the present. Following this brief historical overview, we discuss the current status of public health education in the United States.

Public Health Education: 1914–1939

By the end of the 19th century medical schools had proliferated. There were also many schools of nursing, established by hospitals to provide a source of well-trained labor. However, there was no distinct education or career pattern for public health officers; most were practicing physicians who were called upon to assist with epidemic diseases in times of crisis. It was in this context that staff of the Rockefeller Sanitary Commission attempted to enlist public health officers in the southern United States to

---

[1]Material in the History section of this chapter is abstracted from the commissioned paper prepared for the committee by Elizabeth Fee, Ph.D. The paper appears in its entirety in Appendix D.

aid in a campaign to eradicate hookworm. They found little interest in or dedication to public health, leading Wickliffe Rose, the architect and organizer of the commission, to believe that a new profession was needed, composed of men and women who would devote their entire careers to controlling disease and promoting health at a population level. Three possible approaches for public health education were debated—the engineering or environmental, the sociopolitical, and the biomedical.

Rose enlisted Abraham Flexner in the move to establish education for a separate public health career. On October 16, 1914, Flexner brought together 11 public health representatives and 9 Rockefeller trustees and officers for a meeting. It was decided that there were essentially three categories of public health officers: those with executive authority such as city and state health commissioners; the technical experts in specific fields such as bacteriologists, statisticians, and engineers; and the field workers such as local health officials, factory and food inspectors, and public health nurses.

Rose laid out ideas for a system of public health education centered on a university affiliated, research intensive, scientific school, separate from a medical school, whose graduates would be strategically placed throughout the United States. This central scientific school of public health would be linked to a network of state schools that sent extension agents into the field, and emphasized not only public health education, short courses and extension courses to upgrade the skills of health officers in the field, but also demonstrations of best practices. The plan as implemented, however, focused on research and largely ignored public health practice, administration, public health nursing, and health education. The biomedical side of public health was emphasized to the exclusion of its social and economic context and no attention was given to the political sciences or to the need to plan for social or economic reforms.

The Johns Hopkins University School of Hygiene and Public Health became the first endowed school of public health, opening during the influenza epidemic of 1918. Later, Rockefeller Foundation officials agreed to provide funding for additional schools of public health including ones at Harvard and Toronto. These first schools were well-endowed private institutions that favored persons with medical degrees, had curricula that leaned heavily toward the laboratory sciences, and emphasized infectious diseases. Because the Rockefeller Foundation gave fellowships to medical graduates around the world the schools tended to have an international flavor. Programs of field training were not emphasized. By 1930 these first schools were graduating a small number of individuals with sophisticated scientific education but they were not producing the needed large numbers of public health officers, nurses, and sanitarians.

Public Health Education: 1935 to the Present

Passage of the Social Security Act of 1935 provided a major stimulus to the further development of public health education. Provisions of this act increased funding for the Public Health Service and provided federal grants to the states to assist them in developing their public health services. Federal law now required each state to establish minimal qualifications for health personnel employed using federal assistance, and recommended at least one year of graduate education at an approved school of public health. For the first time, the federal government provided funds, administered through the states, for public health training. Overall, the states budgeted for more than 1,500 public health trainees, and the existing training programs were soon filled to capacity. As a result of the growing demand for public health credentials, several state universities began new schools or divisions of public health and existing schools of public health expanded their enrollments.

In 1936, 10 schools offered public health degrees or certificates requiring at least one year of residence: Johns Hopkins, Harvard, Columbia, Michigan, California at Berkeley, Massachusetts Institute of Technology, Minnesota, Pennsylvania, Wayne State, and Yale (Committee on Professional Education, 1937). By 1938 more than 4,000 people (1,000 of whom were physicians) had received some public health training with funds provided by the federal government through the states. Increased funding and the continuing need for additional public health graduates led many colleges and universities to open public health departments and establish programs offering training courses of a few months' or even a few weeks' duration. Federal training funds were allotted to California, Michigan, Minnesota, Vanderbilt, and North Carolina to develop short courses for the rapid training of public health personnel.

The tremendous push in the late 1930s toward training larger numbers of public health practitioners was also a push toward practical training programs rather than research. Public health departments wanted personnel with one year of public health education: typically, the masters of public health (M.P.H.) generalist degree. If they could not attract public health practitioners holding this credential, they settled for a person with a few months of public health training. Ideally, they also wanted persons who understood practical public health issues rather than scientific specialists with research degrees. Thus, public health education in the 1930s tended to be practically oriented, with considerable emphasis on fields such as public health administration, health education, public health nursing, vital statistics, venereal disease control, and community health services. During this period, too, many schools developed field training programs in local communities where their students could obtain experience in the practical world of public health and prepare for roles within local health departments. The 1930s were thus the prime years of community-based public health education.

The growth of short training programs in public health education continued throughout the war years to meet the demand for physicians, nurses, and sanitarians with at least minimal training in tropical diseases, parasitology, venereal disease control, environmental sanitation, and a variety of infectious diseases. For the burgeoning industrial production areas at home, industrial hygiene was in demand; for areas with military encampments, sanitary engineering and malaria control were urgent concerns.

Schools of public health and public health training programs revamped their educational programs to meet these needs and turned out large numbers of health professionals with a smattering of specialized education in high-priority fields. The research-oriented schools of public health, such as Hopkins and Harvard, maintained their research programs largely by recruiting foreign students—many from Latin America—to staff their laboratory and field programs.

Deans of schools of public health were concerned about the rapid growth of public health education programs and in 1941 organized the Association of Schools of Public Health (ASPH) to promote and improve graduate education for public health professionals. In 1946 the Committee on Professional Education of the American Public Health Association began monitoring the standards of public health education amid complaints that profit-making public health training courses of questionable quality were offering public health degrees by correspondence from faculty who did not even know of their appointment (Shepard, 1948). Demand for minimum adequate standards was increasing. However, a 1950 survey of schools of public health found major difficulties here, too. These schools were overcrowded and under-funded, and lacked key faculty members, classroom and laboratory space, and necessary equipment (Rosenfeld et al., 1953). Under pressure to provide more practical experience, the Deans argued that they needed a 70 percent increase in full-time faculty to expand the applied fields of instruction; they further believed they could double the number of enrolled students if necessary financial support was forthcoming (Rosenfeld et al., 1953).

Given the high demand for public health graduates and the need for schools and programs to train them, it is not surprising that the criteria for accreditation of schools of public health as implemented at mid-century were relatively undemanding by current standards. To become accredited, schools were required to have at least eight full-time professors as well as lecture rooms, seminar rooms, and adequate laboratory facilities; and were to be located close to local public health services that could be used for "observation and criticism." Additionally, these public health services had to be of sufficiently high quality "to make observation fruitful" (Winslow, 1953).

For a few years following World War II the concepts of social medicine, social epidemiology, and the ecology of health achieved prominence. New courses were developed that emphasized the social and economic context of health problems. Schools of public health instituted classes that focused on world population and the food supply; the impact of industry and transportation on health; the impact of cultural, social, and economic forces on health; evaluation of health status; and public health as a community service (Winslow, 1953). At Pittsburgh, Thomas Parran had decided that the curriculum should be organized around "the systematic presentation of illustrative topics which deal with the interrelation of man and his total environment and with the political, economic, and social framework within which the health officer must work" (Blockstein, 1977). Yale's core course on "Principles and Practice of Public Health" was similarly organized around a series of interdisciplinary seminars running throughout the academic year. Winslow commented approvingly that the eleven schools of public health constituted "eleven experimental laboratories in which new pedagogic approaches are constantly being devised" (Winslow, 1953).

The overall impression of the accredited schools of public health in 1950 was that they were doing a good job of preparing public health practitioners through courses and fieldwork, that the numbers of faculty and students were growing, and that curricular and research innovations seemed promising. The main complaints of the schools seemed to be lack of funding to pay faculty, expand space, and purchase equipment.

While schools of public health were concerned about a lack of money, major funding was financing the construction of community hospitals through the Hill-Burton Program, and the National Institutes of Health (NIH) was experiencing rapid growth in research funding. The institutes expanded with enormous increases in financial resources, transferring most of their funds to universities and medical schools in the form of research grants. Grants were awarded based on the decisions of peer review committees composed of non-federal experts in the relevant fields of research. Liberals, conservatives, medical school deans, and researchers were all happy with the system, and members of Congress were pleased to bankroll such a popular and uncontroversial program (Strickland, 1972; Ginzberg and Dutka, 1989).

In this environment schools of public health had to compete with medical schools for research grants in a system dominated by powerful medical school professors. The historic core funders of schools of public health (the major foundations) were turning their interest to building departments of preventive medicine and community medicine within medical schools. Further, increasing political conservatism and the

McCarthy era were having a negative impact on views about public health.

To survive, schools of public health turned to research funding to pay the salaries of additional faculty members, using the rationale that new faculty could spend some of their time teaching and some of their time on funded research. As this strategy was implemented, the following pattern emerged. If a particular department within a school was devoted mainly to teaching or to public health practice, the numbers of faculty stayed stable or gradually declined. If the department was devoted to research, and was reasonably successful at funding that research, the department grew, sometimes at an impressive rate. Even deans who strongly favored teaching and field training over research became unable to resist the pressures that encouraged research over practical training. Available funding, and faculty who were suited by education, experience, and personality to succeed in the research system, shaped the schools of public health and drove their priorities.

Because the system of research funding was not oriented toward field research, public health practice, public health administration, the social sciences, history, politics, law, anthropology, or economics, the laboratory sciences tended to thrive while the practice and other non-quantitative disciplines suffered. The community-based orientation of the 1930s disappeared, and the field training programs virtually ceased to exist.

As faculty withdrew into their laboratories, they further distanced themselves from the problems of the local health departments, which were experiencing increasing difficulty. Federal grants-in-aid to the states for public health programs steadily declined during the 1950s as the total dollar amounts fell from $45 million in 1950 to $33 million in 1959. Given inflation, this represented a dramatic decline in purchasing power (Terris, 1959). Lacking funds, health departments could not afford new people or initiate new programs. Health departments ran underfunded programs with underqualified people who answered to unresponsive bureaucrats.

Between 1947 and 1957 the number of students educated in schools of public health fell by half. Alarmed, Ernest Stebbins of Johns Hopkins and Hugh Leavell of Harvard, representing ASPH, urged Congress to support public health education. They found an especially sympathetic audience in Senator Lister Hill and Representative George M. Rhodes, and in 1958, Congress enacted a two-year emergency program authorizing $1 million a year in federal grants to be divided among the accredited schools of public health.

The First National Conference on Public Health Training in 1958 noted that these funds had provided 1,000 traineeships and had greatly improved morale in public health agencies. The conference further requested appropriations for teaching grants and construction costs for teaching facilities, and urged that faculty salary support be provided for teaching.

Its report concluded with a stirring appeal to value public health education as vital to national defense:

> D' day for disease and death is everyday. The battle line is in our own community. To hold that battle line we must daily depend on specially trained physicians, nurses, biochemists, public health engineers, and other specialists properly organized for the normal protection of the homes, the schools, and the work places of some unidentified city somewhere in America. That city has, today, neither the personnel nor the resources of knowledge necessary to protect it (U.S. DHEW, 1958).

President Dwight Eisenhower signed the Hill-Rhodes Bill, authorizing $1 million annually in formula grants for accredited schools of public health and $2 million annually for five years for project training grants; between 1957 and 1963 the United States Congress appropriated $15 million to support public health trainees. The downward trend in public health enrollments was halted. Between 1960 and 1965 the total number of applicants to schools of public health more than doubled; the number of faculty members increased by 50 percent; the average space occupied increased by 50 percent; and the average income of the schools more than doubled (Fee and Rosenkrantz, 1991).

Following the passage of Medicare and Medicaid legislation in 1965, state health agencies turned to schools of public health to provide the scientific basis for rational decision-making in health services delivery and training for medical care administrators and financial managers. ASPH estimated that 6,220 new positions in medical care administration required graduate-level education (ASPH, 1966). The U.S. Public Health Service provided quick funding to schools of public health to provide short courses in health services administration.

The 1960s brought major progress for the civil rights movement and for President Lyndon B. Johnson's War on Poverty which included the Office of Equal Opportunity (OEO). The OEO helped create 100 neighborhood health centers and the Department of Health, Education, and Welfare (DHEW) supported another 50. A strong environmental movement developed following the publication of Rachel Carson's *Silent Spring* in 1962. In 1970 Earth Day attracted 20 million Americans in demonstrations against assaults on nature; by 1990 Earth Day brought out 200 million participants in 140 countries (McNeil, 2000). The Environmental Protection Agency (EPA) was created and the first Clean Air Act was passed in 1970. Also created during this period were the Occupational Safety and Health Administration (OSHA) and the National Institute of Occupational Safety and Health (NIOSH).

Throughout the 1960s and early 1970s, schools of public health thrived with federal funding available for both teaching programs and research.

In 1960 there were 12 accredited schools of public health in the United States, 8 were added between 1965 and 1975. Between 1965 and 1972, student enrollments again doubled, with the large majority being candidates for the master of public health (M.P.H.) degree. The trend to admit more students who were not physicians, and more students without prior experience in public health continued. In 1946, 61 percent of all students admitted to schools of public health for the M.P.H. were physicians; by 1968–1969 that figure had dropped to only 19 percent of M.P.H. candidates (Hall, 1973).

Along with the growth in the accredited schools of public health came a rapid growth in other forms of public health and health services education. Graduate programs were established in a variety of university departments and schools (e.g., engineering, medicine, nursing, business, social work, education, and communication) offering degrees in such fields as environmental health, health management and administration, nutrition, public health nursing, and health education. Universities were creating popular baccalaureate programs in health administration, environmental engineering, health education, and nutrition. By mid-1970, some 69,000 students were enrolled in various allied health programs (Sheps, 1976). Although 5,000 graduate degrees in public health were awarded each year, approximately half of higher education for public health was occurring outside of accredited schools of public health.

Then, in 1973, President Richard M. Nixon recommended terminating federal support for schools of public health and discontinuing all research training grants, direct traineeships, and fellowships. J. Thomas Grayston of the University of Washington reflected the thoughts of the field when he said:

> the greatest immediate challenge to the School of Public Health and Community Medicine is the uncertainty of federal funding brought about by the administration's announced intention to end, or greatly curtail, federal support for the training of public health manpower, coupled with a similar proposal to decrease support for research training (Grayston, 1974).

The threatened elimination of funding was averted, however, and in 1976 Congress passed the Health Professions Educational Assistance Act (P.L. 94-484), which provided for a number of programs in health professions education. The trend, however, was toward ever more reliance on targeted research funding. Also in 1976 the Milbank Memorial Fund issued its extensive report, *Higher Education for Public Health*, proposing a new structure for the public health educational system—a three tiered structure.

First, schools of public health were to educate people to assume leadership positions. Next, programs in graduate schools would prepare the large number of professionals engaged in providing clearly differentiated specialty services, for example, public health nurses, health educators, and environmental health specialists. Finally baccalaureate programs could provide some of the "trained entry-level personnel" (MMF, 1976). The report identified three core areas of public health on which the schools should focus: epidemiology and biostatistics, social policy and the history and philosophy of public health, and management and organization for public health. In addition, the report recommended that schools should serve as regional resources by helping faculties in medical and other health-related schools to develop teaching programs and research in public health; they should become involved in the operation of community health services; and schools should design their research within a broad framework established by the needs of public health practice.

The report had little impact. Under President Ronald Reagan the pressures intensified. Between 1980 and 1987, spending for health professions' education by the Department of Health and Human Services (DHHS) Bureau of Health Professions declined annually by more than 50 percent from a high of $411,469,000 in 1980 to $189,353,000 in 1987. General purpose traineeship grants to schools of public health dropped from $6,842,000 in 1980 to $2,958,000 in 1987. Project grants for graduate training in public health were funded at $4,949,000 in 1980, but dropped to zero funding in 1982 and remained unfunded through 1987. Curriculum development grants, funded at $7,456,000 in 1980, were not funded at all in 1981 and 1982, but then recovered with funding at $1,740,000 in 1983, then at $2,856,000 in 1984 rising to $9,787,000 in 1987. Grants for graduate programs in health administration were funded at $2,967,000 in 1980, dropped to $726,000 in 1981, and then rose to $1,416,000 in 1982 where funding remained fairly steady, with 1987 levels at $1,482,000 (U.S. DHHS, 1988).

Funding has continued to be problematic for public health education programs and schools of public health. Through the 1990s funding levels remained nearly constant. During that time tuition and other costs continued to increase, resulting in a reduction in the amount of public health professional education actually provided. At the beginning of the 21st century we find a major barrier to workforce development is the "incredibly weak" budget allocated for training (Gebbie, 1999; PHLS, 1999).

Following the events of September 11, 2001, there has been new interest in public health and promises of increased funding. If used wisely, these promised funds will strengthen the public health system through investments in both needed technologies and properly educated and prepared public health professionals. To better understand the future needs of public health education, it is important to examine its current status. The following pages provide a brief overview of public health education in the United States, examine schools of public health in greater detail, and describe progress made since the landmark report *The Future of Public Health* (IOM, 1988).

CURRENT STATUS

Many college graduates who work in public health are educated in other disciplines. For example, of the total public health workforce, nurses make up about 10.9 percent and physicians comprise about 1.3 percent (Center for Health Policy, 2000). The HRSA list of categories of public health occupations includes administrators, professionals, technicians, protective services, paraprofessionals, administrative support, skilled craft workers, and service/maintenance workers. Within these categories fall a number of different kinds of positions (see Appendix E for complete list) including administrative/business professional, public health dental worker, public health veterinarian/animal control specialist, environmental engineering technician, and community outreach/field worker.

Within public health education, the basic public health degree is the M.P.H., while the doctor of public health (Dr.P.H.) is offered for advanced training in public health leadership. There are also individuals working in public health who receive academic degrees (e.g., M.S. and Ph.D.) in public health disciplines such as epidemiology, the biological sciences, biostatistics, environmental health, health services and administration, nutrition, and the social and behavioral sciences. The public health workforce also includes many professionals trained in disciplines such as social work, pharmacy, dentistry, and health and public administration.

Most persons who receive formal education in public health are graduates of one of the 32 accredited schools of public health or of one of the 45 accredited M.P.H. programs. The Council on Education for Public Health (CEPH) is responsible for adopting and applying the criteria that constitute the basis for an accreditation evaluation. In 1998–1999 there were 5,568 graduates from the then 29 accredited schools of public health (ASPH, 2000). The majority of these graduates (61.5 percent) earned an M.P.H. degree, an additional 28.4 percent received a masters degree in some other discipline, and 10.1 percent earned doctoral degrees (ASPH, 2000). According to a survey conducted by Davis and Dandoy (2001), the 45 accredited programs in Community Health and Preventive Medicine (CHPM) and in Community Health Education (CHE) graduate between 700 and 800 master's degree students each year.

There are other programs in which students receive master's level training in public health. These include programs in public administration and affairs, health administration, and M.P.H. programs in schools of medicine. In 1997–1998 an unknown number of the 9,947 graduates of masters degree programs in public administration and affairs (M.P.A.) emphasized public health in their training (NASPAA, 2002). The Association of University

Programs in Health Administration report that in 2000 there were 1,778 graduates who received masters degrees, with some (again an unknown number) of them the M.P.H. and M.S. degrees (AUPHA, 2000). In 1998 of the 125 accredited U.S. medical schools, 36 medical schools offered a combined M.D./M.P.H. degree, and 56 reported that they taught separate required courses on such topics as public health, epidemiology, and biostatistics (Anderson, 1999). Public health workers also may receive undergraduate training from colleges or universities that offer programs in the environmental sciences or in health education and health promotion.

While it is unclear exactly how many public health workers there are in the United States today, it is estimated that about 450,000 people are employed in salaried positions in public health, and an additional 2,850,000 volunteer their services (Center for Health Policy, 2000). This is probably an undercount, according to the Center for Health Policy (2000), because states reporting the number of workers within their jurisdiction almost never include information about public health workers found in non-governmental and community partner agencies. Additionally, limited information is obtained regarding the numbers of volunteers and salaried staff in voluntary agencies. Persons who graduate with training in public health are, however, only a small portion of the public health workforce. Nationally, it has been estimated that 80 percent of public health workers lack specific public health training (CDC, 2001c) and only 22 percent of chief executives of local health departments have graduate degrees in public health (Turnock, 2001).

Schools of Public Health

Schools of public health vary in many ways including size, organization, and degrees offered All schools offer courses in the five areas identified as core to public health: biostatistics, epidemiology, environmental health sciences, health services administration, and social and behavioral sciences. The extent and breadth of offerings within these categories varies, however. In addition, schools offer courses in a number of other areas including nutrition, biomedical and laboratory sciences, disease control, genetics, and much more (please see Appendix A).

Progress in Schools of Public Health

In 1988 the Institute of Medicine (IOM) report, *The Future of Public Health,* described the field of public health as being in disarray (IOM, 1988). The focus of that report was on public health practice but it did have a number of recommendations for schools of public health. These recommendations called for

- new linkages between public health schools and programs, and public health agencies at the federal, state, and local levels;
- the development of new training opportunities for professionals who are already practicing in public health;
- development of new relationships within universities between public health schools and programs and other professional schools and departments;
- the conduct of a wide range of research that includes basic and applied research and research on program evaluation and implementation;
- more extensive approaches to education that encompass the full scope of public health practice; and
- strengthening the knowledge base in the areas of international health and the health of minority groups.

The report also urged schools of public health to serve as resources to government at all levels in the development of public health policy. In summary, the task defined by the IOM report was "to assist the schools in developing a greater emphasis on public health practice and to equip them to train personnel with the breadth of knowledge that matches the scope of public health" (IOM, 1988). The following describes the progress schools of public health have made in implementing the IOM report recommendations.

Strengthening the link with public health practice. Fineberg and colleagues (1994) identify the 1988 IOM report's insistence "that professional education be grounded in 'real world' public health" as the most influential recommendation in the report. This recommendation generated a number of initiatives aimed at establishing a closer relationship between schools of public health and public health practice. One of the first efforts following the IOM report was a collaborative study by the Johns Hopkins School of Hygiene and Public Health and the ASPH (funded by HRSA and CDC in 1989) to define the essential elements of the profession of public health. Public health practitioners and faculty from the schools of public health were brought together in the Public Health Faculty/Agency Forum, issuing a report in 1991 that emphasized:

- public health education based upon universal competencies of public health practice; and
- cooperation between schools of public health and public health agencies, including supervised practica for students (Fineberg et al., 1994).

The forum also recommended changing accreditation criteria to emphasize the practice of public health. In response, CEPH revised accreditation criteria to include a required practicum experience.

In 1991 the Council on Linkages Between Academia and Public Health Practice was established to "promote activities that link public health academic programs with the practice community through refining and implementing the forum recommendations" (Eisen et al., 1994). The Council, which includes representatives from national public health academic institutions and practice organizations, has initiated many efforts to enhance academic/practice collaboration. These include demonstration programs that examine academic/practice linkage approaches (Bialek, 2001), a national public health practice research agenda (Conrad, 2000), and a set of core competencies for public health professionals. The core competencies are organized around three job categories—front line staff, senior level staff, and supervisory management staff (Council on Linkages, 2001).

Schools of public health also have undertaken new initiatives to increase practice linkages. One of these is community-based participatory research, a research approach that involves all stakeholders in each aspect of a study designed to evaluate the application and impact of new discoveries aimed at improving the health of a defined population. This approach to research is discussed in greater detail in Chapter 3. It requires active partnerships between the community and researchers who may or may not be members of that community. Partnerships and coalitions are important in developing prevention and health promotion programs or research today, because no single agency has the resources, access, and trust relationships to address the wide range of community determinants of public health problems (Green et al., 2001).

Other approaches to strengthening ties between schools of public health and public health practice were reported in a survey of schools of public health. The committee conducted a survey of schools of public health (Appendix B) that listed recommendations from *The Future of Public Health* (IOM, 1988) and asked schools to indicate what they had done in response. The survey was mailed by ASPH in February 2002 to all accredited schools. Of the then 31 accredited schools of public health, 25 responded to the survey, a response rate of 80.6 percent (see Table 2-1 for list of respondents).

One key recommendation in the 1988 report concerned linkages with state and local health departments, which are important to strengthening ties with the practice community. Each of the respondent schools indicated that at least some, and in some instances many, of their faculty have professional working relationships with state or local health departments or both. Their activities include conducting requested research projects, providing technical assistance, serving as the local epidemiologist or health officer, providing staff development or training, or serving on professional advisory committees. Major barriers to student involvement in

TABLE 2-1   Respondent Schools of Public Health ($n = 25$)

Boston University	University at Albany	University of Michigan
Emory University	(SUNY)	University of Minnesota
Harvard University	University of California,	University of North
Johns Hopkins	Berkeley	Carolina, Chapel Hill
Ohio State University	University of California,	University of Oklahoma
Saint Louis University	Los Angeles	University of Pittsburgh
San Diego State	University of Iowa	University of South
University	University of	Carolina
Texas A&M University	Massachusetts	University of Texas,
Tulane University	University of Medicine	Houston
University of Alabama,	and Dentistry of	University of Washington
Birmingham	New Jersey	Yale University

activities with state and local health agencies were identified as lack of financial support and geographical distance from the health department.

The survey also asked about the importance of practice experience as criteria for admission of student applicants or in the faculty hiring process. For faculty recruitment, prior practice experience was rated very important or important by about one-third (32 percent) of the respondent schools while for student admission about one-half or 52 percent of schools rated prior experience very important or important.

Ties between schools of public health and the practice communities have been strengthened, but barriers remain. Foremost among the barriers is a lack of funding and incentives for such activities. As discussed earlier, schools of public health obtain most of their funding primarily through research grants and contracts, because federal support for teaching and practice activities has declined enormously during the past two decades and has not been replaced by state or private sources of funding. Additionally, the incentive and reward structure for faculty tenure and promotion is weighted heavily toward research and publication; teaching and practice activities carry comparatively little weight.

Another 1988 recommendation for linking schools to practice is for schools to participate in policy development. The survey asked schools to indicate how they fulfill their potential role as significant resources to government at all levels in the development of public health policy as well as barriers to engaging in this role. The vast majority of schools that responded have faculty who engage in numerous policy development activities as reflected in Table 2-2.

New training opportunities.   *The Future of Public Health* (IOM, 1988) recommended that schools of public health improve their educational approaches for the practicing public health workforce through short courses and continuing education. Currently, all accredited schools of public health

TABLE 2-2   Number and Percent of Schools Engaged in State
Governmental Activities During the Past Five Years ($n = 25$)

	Policy Development for Legislative Body	Public Health Advocacy with State Government	Public Health Advocacy with Local Government	Research Requested by State Policy-makers	Research Requested by Local Policy-makers	Public Health Workforce Development
Number	23	23	22	23	21	24
Percent	92	92	88	92	84	96

offer continuing education for public health professionals, as do the accredited programs. The overarching goal of continuing professional education is to educate and support public health professionals through enhancement of their knowledge and skills in public health practice, theory, research, and policy. Continuing education is an essential component of any career, according to Gordon and McFarlane (1996), and all schools and practice agencies should develop appropriate support systems for relevant continuing education for public health practitioners.

One approach to continuing education is to offer yearly conferences or workshops on specific topics. These programs can be sponsored by a college or university or in partnership with public health programs, agencies, or associations. They usually carry continuing education credits to meet the re-certification needs of the anticipated audience. Certificate programs are another approach to educating those currently working in public health. About one-third of the accredited schools of public health currently offer certificate programs. Standards for admission and completion vary across schools. Certificate programs may be general and emphasize core public health concepts from the five core content areas taught in M.P.H. programs, that is, epidemiology, biostatistics, environmental health sciences, health services administration, and social and behavioral sciences. Others focus on a specific content area such as international health, environmental health, occupational health, injury control, health policy, or health administration.

The CDC Graduate Certificate Program (GCP)—a program no longer funded—was a prime example of certificate programs. It was designed for CDC field officers, state health department personnel, and selected others with at least three to five years of experience in public health practice. The program allowed CDC Public Health Advisors working in state and local health departments to earn a graduate certificate in public health and was available from one of four accredited schools of public health: Tulane University School of Public Health and Tropical Medicine, Emory University Rollins School of Public Health, Johns Hopkins University

Bloomberg School of Public Health, and University of Washington School of Public Health and Community Medicine.

Academic institutions (including schools of public health) also offer summer institutes and courses. Subjects encompassed range from basic biostatistics, epidemiology, and Geographic Information Systems (GIS) applications, to management and administration for middle to senior managers. Such programs can vary in length from a single one-day course to week-long offerings. Another approach to traditional continuing education programs, as described by Halverson and colleagues (1997), involves the creation of masters- and doctoral-level executive programs that minimize time lost from work through use of distance learning teaching methods. By enabling workers to continue in their work responsibilities while completing self-paced coursework, this approach reduces the burden overworked and understaffed agencies feel as their staff members participate in educational programs.

The introduction of Web-based tools for education is producing a major change in the way schools and colleges conduct classes, particularly in the area of continuing education. The use of such technology is referred to as *distance learning* (Riegelman and Persily, 2001). This development builds upon more than two decades of computer networking activities (e.g., e-mail and bulletin board systems), and the increased availability of the Internet has produced phenomenal growth in the extent and scope of online education. Distance learning today has become an important alternative to traditional methods of education, because the existing technology has the potential to facilitate complicated distance learning environments and highly structured learning methods (Mattheos et al., 2001). The Public Health Training Network (PHTN) is an example of successful promotion of distance learning. This network has linked nearly one million people to training on a wide range of subjects in a variety of formats: print-based self-instruction, interactive multimedia, videotapes, two-way audio conferences, and interactive satellite videoconferences (CDC, 2001b).

Links with other departments and schools. *The Future of Public Health* (IOM, 1988) recommended that schools of public health develop new relationships with other schools and departments both within their universities as well as with other institutions of higher learning. Such collaboration is taking place, according to survey data. For example, 96 percent of reporting schools ($n = 24$) indicated that their public health students could take courses in schools of medicine that would count toward their degree, as did 64 percent ($n = 16$) for courses in nursing, 44 percent ($n = 11$) in dentistry, 68 percent ($n = 17$) in law, and 72 percent ($n = 18$) in social work. Fifty-six percent ($n = 14$) of responding schools reported that students "often" avail themselves of these opportunities in other schools and departments and 28 percent responded "sometimes."

Research. "[R]esearch in schools of public health should range from basic research in fields related to public health, through applied research and development, to program evaluation and implementation research" (IOM, 1988). To describe the range of research conducted in schools of public health the committee survey asked each school to estimate the percentage of research undertaken at the school that the respondent would characterize as:

- basic or fundamental research, that is, research conducted for the purpose of advancing our knowledge;
- applied research, that is, research designed to use the results of other research (e.g., basic research) to solve real world problems;
- translational research, that is, research on approaches for translating results of other types of research to community use; or
- evaluative research, that is, the use of scientific methods to assess the effectiveness of a program or initiative.

Among respondent schools the distribution of the types of research undertaken varied greatly. On average, applied research was reported most often (35 percent mean, range of 10–60 percent), followed by basic research (27 percent mean, range of 0–70 percent), evaluative research (20 percent mean, range of 1–50 percent), and translational research (17 percent mean, range 0–30 percent).

Broadening the scope of public health education. The 1988 IOM report recommended that schools of public health provide an opportunity to learn the entire range of skills and knowledge necessary for public health practice. Recent efforts to encompass a broad scope of education have focused on identifying basic competencies in public health and on developing curricula that teach the information and skills necessary to meet those competencies. The CDC Office of Workforce Policy and Planning (CDC, 2001c) has developed a table of public health competency sets (Appendix F). One of these is a set of core competencies developed by the Council on Linkages Between Academia and Public Health Practice (Council on Linkages, 2001). The ASPH has endorsed the Council on Linkages competencies and plans to develop complementary competencies for M.P.H. students.

One competency area relates to cultural competence. The committee survey of schools of public health requested respondents to indicate courses that they offer students in cultural or international health as well as other selected areas. Table 2-3 presents their responses.

TABLE 2-3 Number and Percent of Responding Schools Offerings
Courses in Selected Areas (*n* = 25)

	Cultural Com- petencies	Ethics	Health Disparities	Social Justice	Human Rights	International/ Global Health	Social Epidemi- ology
Number	16	22	19	17	13	18	15
Percent	64	88	76	68	52	72	60

The final question on the committee survey of schools of public health asked for input on identifying the most important challenges and opportunities facing schools of public health and M.P.H. programs over the next 10 years. The following summarizes responses to this question.

Survey responses identifying challenges and opportunities. According to respondents, public health as a profession is not well defined. Lack of clear definition is one reason the public does not understand the field. Raising public awareness of public health's contributions to health and quality of life is important. Such awareness would help assure adequate support for public health programs. Lack of support and funding was a *major* issue identified frequently. Respondents indicated that increased funding is needed to support students and workforce development, and is critical to maintaining stable support for key academic programs including teaching. The major revenue source for schools of public health (i.e., external research funding) is seen as incongruent with the teaching mission and results in devaluing teaching and educational activities.

Respondents indicated that the changing environment and ever-widening scope of public health requires collaboration and partnerships with other disciplines. Additionally, within the field, schools need to build strong relationships among academia, scientists, and the professional practice community, thereby allowing each to benefit from the assets of the others.

Education and training issues were identified by numerous respondents. As one person wrote, "Public health is no different than other academic programs in that we tend to produce graduates for yesterday's workplace and yesterday's problems. Producing M.P.H. graduates responsive to what is needed today requires an understanding of the driving forces that affect public health practice and the public health workforce." Respondents indicated that major needs include understanding that multiple factors influence health and that public health issues require societal change as well as changes in individual behavior for risk reduction. One respondent indicated that the primary goal of schools of public health should be to train the next generation of leaders as public health scientists and public health professionals, stating that "Research informs practice and policy. Leadership guides them all." The need for competencies in public health was mentioned several times. Other educational or training issues included:

- Education at the M.P.H. level should be comprehensive, integrated, and broad-based to support the need for general public health preparedness, necessary for such things as bioterrorism preparedness.
- M.P.H. programs need to be redesigned to permit greater flexibility in the development of clusters of skills and competencies in response to the rapidly changing public health environment.
- Baccalaureate training in schools would provide a vehicle for attracting a new cadre of students into public health.
- There is a need for opportunities for training in non-degree programs for part-time and mid-career students, and for increased distance learning programs.
- There is a need for more practical experience for graduates.

Faculty issues were also addressed. Respondents indicated the need to recruit minority faculty to achieve diversity, that it was difficult to recruit faculty in specific disciplines such as biostatistics and epidemiology, and that it is necessary to maintain and improve faculty salary levels to be competitive with other sectors.

Another issue identified as important was building the public health infrastructure. Some respondents indicated that there should be national attention and standards for trained personnel, along with funding to meet those standards. Respondents indicated that schools should be expected to be a resource to provide training and to meet these standards and that a lack of standards and funding results in an inadequately prepared public health workforce. It was suggested that certification or credentialing of public health professionals is an important issue. One person suggested that certification might result in more uniform and rigorous programs to address core content needs. It was proposed that schools assist in the accreditation process for local departments of health by helping them meet their continuing education needs.

Respondents also indicated that the emphasis of public health research must be reviewed periodically. More prevention research is needed, including increased federal interest in prevention research. Schools of public health must more effectively promote prevention as a powerful means of health protection. Public health must find new approaches to reach the public on a level that effectively encourages primary prevention and enables individuals to change known risk behaviors to healthy behaviors. There should be increased emphasis on partnerships to develop viable research programs. Understanding and addressing the determinants of ethnic and racial health disparities is an important research focus.

It was suggested that new monies flowing into public health for bioterrorism response should be used to help build the infrastructure. Finally, respondents identified, but did not elaborate on, the following challenges:

- Globalizaation
- Re-emerging infections
- Human genome
- Quality of health care
- Un- and under-insured populations
- Population aging

SUMMARY

The establishment of the Johns Hopkins University School of Hygiene and Public Health in 1918 marked the beginning of public health education in a school dedicated to the field. There are currently 32 accredited schools of public health and 45 accredited community health programs. The Council on Education for Public Health estimates that the total number of accredited schools and programs may well double within the next 10 years and that the most dramatic growth is occurring outside the established schools of public health. Many of the nation's accredited medical schools now have operational M.P.H. programs or are currently developing a graduate public health degree program (Evans, 2002). New specializations are emerging such as human genetics, management of clinical trials, and public health informatics. Many schools and competing organizations are involved in distance learning programs that offer the possibility of fulfilling the long-recognized need to bring public health education to the homes and offices of the public health workforce. The Internet also offers the possibility of bringing public health education to populations across the country and around the world; indeed, health information sites are among the most popular and frequently visited of all Web applications.

Previous efforts to design truly effective systems of public health education generally foundered because of a lack of political will, public disinterest, or a paucity of funds. Since September 11, 2001, however, the context has changed dramatically. With public health rising high on the national agenda and an abundance of funds being promised, perhaps there is now an opportunity, as there has not been for a very long time, to shape a future system of public health education that addresses the problems that have been so often described and analyzed.

3

The Future of Public Health Education

Public health in the United States in the early 1900s focused on improving sanitation, controlling infectious diseases, assuring the safety of the food and water supply, and providing immunizations to children with a workforce composed mostly of physicians, nurses, and biological scientists (Brandt and Gardner, 2000; Garrett, 2000; Mullan, 2000). Today's public health challenges are much broader. *Healthy People 2010* lays out a broad agenda for public health efforts aimed at increasing health-related quality of life and eliminating health disparities (U.S. DHHS, 2000). Koplan and Fleming (2000) outline 10 challenges for public health that include cleaning up the environment, eliminating health disparities, wisely using new scientific knowledge and technology, attending to children's physical and emotional development, and aging healthily. Numerous authors have highlighted the importance of public health in addressing the effects of globalization (Lee, 2000; McMichael and Beaglehole, 2000; Barks-Ruggles, 2001; Kickbusch and Buse, 2001) and the impacts of an aging and increasingly diverse society (Brownson and Kreuter, 1997; Butler, 1997; Koplan and Fleming, 2000; Turnock, 2001).

These complex problems require multi-faceted public health actions based on an ecological approach to problem solving. Such an approach requires a well-educated interdisciplinary cadre of public health professionals who focus on population health and understand the multiple determinants that affect health. A cadre of professionals who also understand that successful interventions require understanding not only of the effects of biology and behavior, but also the social, environmental, and economic contexts within which populations exist. A cadre of professionals who understand that public health research must focus not only on secondary prevention and risk factor analysis, but also on evaluation of public health systems, on practice approaches and interventions, and on effective collaborations and partnerships with diverse communities.

Public health professionals of the future will need to understand and be able to use the new information systems that provide the data upon which public health research and practice is based. They will need to be able to communicate with diverse populations, to understand the issues, concerns, and needs of these groups in order to work collaboratively to improve population health. Public health professionals must have the skills and competencies necessary to engage in public health practice at many levels: leadership, management, and supervisory.

The committee reaffirms the importance of the traditional core public health areas of epidemiology, biostatistics, environmental health, health services administration, and social and behavioral sciences. However, the committee believes that public health professionals will be better prepared to address the major health problems and challenges facing society if they achieve competency in the following eight content areas: informatics, genomics, communication, cultural competence, community-based participatory research, global health, policy and law, and public health ethics. These eight areas are now and will continue to be significant to public health and public health education in programs and schools of public health for some time to come. These areas are natural outgrowths of the traditional core public health sciences as they have evolved in response to ongoing social, economic, technological, and demographic changes. For example, community-based participatory research (CBPR) is a contemporary approach to research that has its roots in the public health sciences of epidemiology and biostatistics, enriched by emerging community knowledge from the social and behavioral sciences.

The following sections of this chapter provide an in-depth examination of these eight areas of critical importance to public health education in the 21st century. Competency in each of these areas will enable public health professionals to better function within the ecological model (discussed in Chapter 1), thereby contributing effectively to programs, policies, and research designed to improve the health of the public. For each of these areas we provide a brief definition and description, explore why each is important to public health, examine the minimum level of knowledge or understanding public health professionals should have about each area, and highlight potential ethical issues.

INFORMATICS

Capacity to perform the public health functions specified in *The Future of Public Health* (IOM, 1988), namely, assessment, policy development and assurance, is principally dependent upon information. For example, *assessment* involves the collection, analysis, interpretation, and communication of information. Currently, this information comes from a wide variety of sources with attendant problems of fragmentation, lack of standardization, and redundancy. *Policy development* also is dependent upon current and reliable information and the ability to manipulate and display this information so that it is meaningful to those who make decisions about public health. *Assurance* requires information about access to health care services based upon community needs, which is monitored with community-level data. With increasing accessibility to more and more data, public health practitioners and researchers will find that a basic understanding of informatics, the use of informatics tools, and interaction with informaticians are essential to carrying out these functions.

Public health informatics is defined as the systematic application of information, computer science, and technology to public health practice and learning (Yasnoff et al., 2000). Its scope includes the conceptualization, design, development, deployment, refinement, maintenance, and evaluation of communication, surveillance, and information systems relevant to public health. Public health informatics involves more than automating existing activities; it enables the redesign of systems using approaches that were previously impractical or not even contemplated.

Public health informatics has immense potential not only to improve current public health practice, but to transform present-day capacity. The September 11, 2001, terrorist attack on the World Trade Center in New York City and the following anthrax distribution and deaths dramatically exemplifies the need for transformation and improvement. Of crucial importance is the collection of real time data on the occurrence of suspicious respiratory syndromes (e.g., possible early anthrax, plague, smallpox, or tularemia) to generate a more rapid and effective public health response (Rotz et al., 2000). For early response to bioterrorism, new data sources, such as emergency room, over-the-counter pharmacy data, absentee or 911 call data may supply potentially essential information. This type of surveillance will require an integrated approach, standardization, closer integration of public health and the health care system, and the timely capture of data.

Improved surveillance systems are likely to tax the public health system's capacity to process the growing quantity of health data required for public health improvement. Progressively, state and local governments are collecting and disseminating health status data at greater levels of detail, the number of reportable diseases is enlarging, and new developments in electronic laboratory reporting systems and electronic medical record systems will also increase the volume of data available to the public health system. Informatics methods and applications, such as decision support and expert systems, modeling and simulation techniques, can help public health face this challenge by providing increased capacity to handle, analyze, and act on data that is likely to increase during the coming years.

Health promotion and disease prevention is another aspect of public health that can be dramatically transformed by informatics. Methods and applications ranging from interactive guideline dissemination, preventive care reminders linked to the electronic medical record, computerized health risk assessments, and tailored messages can help health promotion and disease prevention interventions become more effective than ever before. Web-based systems are offering new strategies in health education. Applications can provide decision support for consumers, focusing on personalized goal setting, feedback regarding progress toward goals, and social support. Consumers of health care and patients managing chronic health conditions can make use of electronic portals to share coping strategies, provide emotional support, and exchange information on relevant health Websites.

Consumer health informatics has been defined as the field of biomedical informatics that is concerned with this area. Informatics methods and applications are stimulating research and development in the use of information and communication technologies. In the broadest sense, consumer health informatics involves (1) analyzing, formalizing, and modeling consumer preferences and information needs; (2) developing methods to integrate these into information management in health promotion, clinical, educational, and research activities; (3) investigating the effectiveness and efficacy of computerized information, telecommunication, and network systems for consumers in relation to their participation in health and health care related activities; and (4) studying the effects of these systems on public health, the patient-professional relationship, and society.

It is both inevitable and desirable that health promotion and disease prevention interventions become more available electronically, empowering consumers with enhanced control over their health. Public health professionals working to ensure the public's health can help consumers by developing and increasing the availability of health-promoting technology based applications, and by safeguarding the confidentiality and security of the health data to which consumers are likely to be electronically exposed.

A critical challenge for public health informatics is to educate the public health workforce in computing and communication technology applicable to public health activities. Some level of informatics training for both new and existing public health workers is essential. Just as every public health professional needs basic knowledge of epidemiology, a basic understanding of public health informatics is critical for effective practice in the information age (Yasnoff et al., 2000). The extent to which information transforms the practice of public health will be determined, in large part, by the willingness of public health leaders to recognize the need for informatics training. Several initiatives have been undertaken recently to promote this recognition.

The American Medical Informatics Association (AMIA) 2001 Spring Congress brought together the public health and informatics communities to develop a national agenda for public health informatics (PHI). The consensus of the session devoted to the topic of informatics training for the public health workforce was that the public health workforce urgently needed informatics knowledge and skills that could best be provided by a spectrum of educational programs (Yasnoff et al., 2001). Other, more detailed recommendations were to establish new and strengthen existing academic programs in PHI, develop a national competency-based continuing education program in PHI, adapt the American Association of Medical Colleges (AAMC) medical school informatics objectives to PHI, and support the Centers for Disease Control and Prevention (CDC) and other efforts to develop core competencies in PHI.

CDC has established the Public Health Informatics Competencies Working Group to develop core competencies in public health informatics within the broader context of the Global and National Implementation Plan for Public Health Workforce Development with an initial focus on developing informatics competencies for the existing U.S. public health workforce. As of this writing, a document has been drafted identifying competencies for the three workforce segments defined by the Council on Linkages. Competencies are divided into two general classes. The first class includes competencies related to the use of information and computer sciences and technology to increase one's individual effectiveness as a public health professional. Examples of these competencies include:

- electronic communication (use of IT tools for the full range of electronic communication appropriate to one's programmatic area);
- on-line information access (use of IT tools to identify, locate, access, assess, and appropriately interpret and use on-line public health-related information and data);
- data and system protection (application of relevant procedures to ensure that confidential information is appropriately protected);
- distance learning (use of distance-learning technologies to support life-long learning); and
- strategic use of IT to promote health (use of IT as a strategic tool to promote public health).

The second class of competencies is related to the development, deployment, and maintenance of information systems to improve the effectiveness of the public health enterprise.

CDC also has made initial efforts to develop needed education programs through the public health informatics fellowship, a public health informatics course, and a cooperative effort with the National Library of Medicine to help train public health workers in the effective use of the information resources available on the Internet.

Most current public health workers, lacking the knowledge and skills necessary to apply information and science technology, are unable to take advantage of its potential to enhance and facilitate public health activities (Lasker et al., 1995). For general public health practitioners, it may be adequate to have a basic understanding of well-established processes used in information systems development as well as an understanding of the roles public health practitioners should play in those processes. For public health professionals wishing to specialize, a higher-level proficiency in informatics is needed as it relates to project management; organizational behavior and management, information and knowledge development (data standards, security, privacy, and confidentiality); systems development, planning, and procurement; fundamental aspects of IT research, decision-making, and outcomes research. Facilitating advanced public health applications of information technology will require a cadre of public health professionals with advanced informatics training in addition to significant improvements in the basic technology literacy of the general workforce in public health, and ongoing training to continuously update information skills (Lasker et al., 1995).

Ideally, public health informatics education would include developing degree and certificate granting programs, and instructional courses for public health agencies and collaborators. Informatics training is becoming increasingly widespread, although training varies by institution, some offering graduate degrees or certificates in informatics, others a course for graduate credit or continuing education. Several graduate programs in public health already offer an informatics course, and a few are offering degrees specializing in informatics. Efforts to provide informatics training through distance education also are increasing. The Association of Schools of Public Health (ASPH) has sponsored conferences on public health informatics and distance learning that focused on how people and technology can work together to positively impact public health practice. The User Liaison Program (ULP) of the Agency for Healthcare Research and Quality (AHRQ) has broadcast a Web-assisted audio teleconference series via the World Wide Web and telephone designed to help state and local policy makers make policy decisions and allocate resources related to health care informatics. Expansion of these and other efforts are important to provide the public health informatics education for the current and future public health workforce.

Research efforts are also required to investigate the applicability of information science and technology to public health. Public health informatics research is essential to help set priorities for resources and ensure that new ideas are adequately tested prior to implementation. Academic researchers in public health have important roles to perform at the cross-roads between informatics and public health. The focus of public health on prevention, communities, surveillance, and longitudinal analysis introduces unique opportunities for informatics research (Yasnoff et al., 2001). Academic researchers in public health possess the expertise to help guide a research agenda and priorities for allocation of resources that concentrate on unique public health concerns that could have a substantial impact on public health practice. Contributions of this expertise to multidisciplinary research collaborations can increase the chances that this complex research will be successful and relevant to public health.

Specific research agenda items suggested at the American Medication Informatics 2001 Spring Congress include assessing informatics tools as they relate to real-time data acquisition; data mining for population data; assessing informatics tools for managing temporal, spatial, or multilevel data; developing methods of measuring the cost of informatics and the benefit that accrues from its use; determining the informatics aspects of a preventive health record for the community; studying the ethical issues needed to guide confidentiality policy; and determining the value and impact of the use of uniform coding and common clinical vocabulary on public health activities (Yasnoff et al., 2001). Uniform coding, the use of existing national standards, and identifying priorities for the development of new data standards are of great importance to public health informatics research. Representation in collaborations such as the Public Health Data Standards Consortium (PHDSC) is yet another significant role for public health academic researchers.

Cross-fertilization between government and academia and local and state agencies can stimulate interest and capacity to support new innovations in the use of technology in public health practice. An example initiated by CDC is the national network of Centers for Public Health Preparedness (CPHP) to strengthen bioterrorism and emergency preparedness at the front lines by linking academic expertise and assets to state and local health agency needs. A number of centers are currently providing public health professionals with connections to online resources and the opportunities to learn technology-based skills that can be applied in their work setting.

The critical challenge of educating the public health workforce in computing and communication technology applicable to public health activities will require collaborative action involving those working in the field; professional associations; local, state, and federal government agencies; library and information service providers; and programs and schools of public health.

We live in an information age that is transforming the ways in which we engage in actions to improve health. Public health professionals of the 21st century must learn about public health informatics and understand how this science contributes to the core functions of assessment, policy development, and assurance activities. Public health professionals must be prepared to understand and use these new information technologies to most effectively work to improve the health of the public. Another major area of scientific and technological development is the field of genomics. The following section discusses this important area.

GENOMICS

We have entered an era in which the genetic factors in common and complex diseases are becoming well understood and in which important new preventive and therapeutic approaches will derive from improved understanding of genetics and genomics. Research in *genetics*—the study of single genes and their functions and effects—has provided increasingly detailed information about both the basic biology and the phenotypic manifestations of several disorders that are caused by abnormality in the number of chromosomes present (such as Down syndrome, Trisomy 18 and Turner syndrome). Such also has been the case in a somewhat larger number of disorders caused by deletions or additions of fairly large segments of chromosomes (such as "cri-du-chat" syndrome and 22q11 deletion syndrome), and for several thousand conditions caused by mutations in single genes (such as cystic fibrosis, sickle cell disease, Tay-Sachs disease, hereditary hemochromatosis, Marfan syndrome, Prader-Willi syndrome, and hereditary hemorrhagic telangiectasia). Having one of these thousands of disorders often has significant impact on the health, and even life, of an affected individual and, frequently, on other family members.

Certain of these "chromosomal" or "single-gene" conditions (such as Down syndrome and hemochromatosis) are relatively common in the general population in the United States, but even they occur in only one of several hundred individuals. Others (such as sickle cell disease among African Americans and Tay-Sachs disease among Ashkenazi Jews), while rare in the general population, are more common in specific population groups. Nonetheless, the overall frequency of chromosomal and single-gene conditions as a group is low in the general population in the United States. Moreover, there have been relatively few effective therapeutic interventions for chromosomal and single-gene conditions. Because of the relative rarity of chromosomal and single-gene conditions and the limited effective therapeutic strategies for them, genetics has not played a significant role in most individuals' health care, and therefore, genetics has been a relatively minor part of medicine.

Genetics has traditionally played an even smaller role in public health. Not only has it been relevant to the health of relatively few people, but there have been almost no effective preventive strategies for chromosomal and single-gene conditions. The major exception to this has been newborn screening (prenatal genetic screening has also been widely practiced; however, it differs importantly from newborn screening in that it is used early in pregnancy to detect major chromosomal abnormalities and birth defects). In the almost 40 years since its inception, newborn screening has become an important public health activity in all states of the United States and in many other developed countries.

However, genetics has now evolved into *genomics*, the study of the entire human genome—the approximately 35,000 genes that humans possess. Because genomics encompasses not only the actions of single genes but also the interactions of multiple genes with each other and with the environment, genomics has far wider applicability to health and disease than does genetics alone. With the arrival of the era in which we will have the ability to understand gene-environment interactions comes not only the era of genomic medicine, but of genomics-based public health. Understanding genomics, therefore, is essential for an effective public health workforce.

Consider for instance, Table 3-1, which is based upon preliminary figures from the CDC, and shows the 10 leading causes of mortality in the United States in 2000. Genetic factors play a significant causative role in at least 9 of these 10 leading causes of morbidity in the United States—injury is the only possible exception. (However, this may hold true for injuries; since genetic factors often play a significant role in the individual host's response to trauma, they play a significant role in determining whether a specific injury proves fatal to a specific person.)

Although it has been widely known that genetic factors played a role in conditions like those in Table 3-1, until recently the precise identity of those factors was not known. However, we have entered an era in which we are rapidly identifying these factors. Moreover, we also are beginning to be able to design new effective therapeutic and preventive strategies based upon this knowledge.

One might assume that it is only in the United States and other developed countries that genomics is on the brink of making major contributions to health. That is not the case. A recent report on genomics and world health (WHO, 2002) points out that genetic research has the potential to lead to major advances in combating such important global diseases as tuberculosis, malaria, and HIV/AIDS in the developing world *within the next three to five years.*

If understanding genomics is essential to today's and tomorrow's public health workforce, what is the appropriate level of understanding of genomics that programs and schools of public health should endeavor

TABLE 3-1   Causes of Death in the United States, 2000

	Cause of Death	Percentage of All U.S. Deaths
1	Heart disease	29.5%
2	Cancer	22.9%
3	Cerebrovascular diseases	6.9%
4	Chronic lower respiratory diseases	5.1%
5	Injury	3.9%
6	Diabetes	2.9%
7	Pneumonia/influenza	2.8%
8	Alzheimer disease	2.0%
9	Renal disease	1.6%
10	Septicemia	1.3%

Based on preliminary data. Derived from information obtained on http://www.cdc.gov/nchs/data/nvsr/nvsr49/nvsr49_12.pdf.

to provide to their students? All public health students should learn to "think genomically," to be able to apply an understanding of genomics to a variety of public health issues. Two groups have provided valuable considerations of "core competencies" in genomics and genetics that help pinpoint what this might mean in terms of public health education.

The National Coalition for Health Professional Education in Genetics, a coalition of more than 120 health professional organizations, has promulgated a set of competencies in genetics and genomics (Jenkins et al., 2001). The CDC also convened an interdisciplinary group that produced a set of competencies in genetics and genomics specific to the public health workforce (CDC, 2001d). These competencies supply a particularly worthwhile set of guideposts for public health education. The competencies are recommended for all public health professionals, and thus one might consider these the competencies that programs and schools of public health should provide all of their students. These are the abilities to:

• apply the basic public health sciences, (including behavioral and social sciences, biostatistics, epidemiology, informatics, and environmental health) to genomic issues and studies and genetic testing, using the genomic vocabulary to attain the goal of disease prevention;
• identify ethical and medical limitations to genetic testing, including uses that don't benefit the individual;
• maintain up-to-date knowledge on the development of genetic advances and technologies relevant to an individual in his/her specialty or field of expertise and learn the uses of genomics as a tool for achieving public health goals related to that person's field or area of practice;
• identify the role of cultural, social, behavioral, environmental, and genetic factors in the development of disease, in disease prevention, and

in health promoting behaviors; and the impact of these factors on medical service organization and delivery of services to maximize wellness and prevent disease;

- participate in strategic policy planning and development related to genetic testing or genomic programs;
- collaborate with existing and emerging health agencies and organizations, and academic, research, private, and commercial enterprises, including genomic-related businesses, agencies and organizations and community partnerships to identify and solve genomic-related problems;
- participate in the evaluation of program effectiveness, accessibility, cost-benefit, cost effectiveness, and quality of personal and population-based genomic services in public health; and
- develop protocols to ensure informed consent and human subject protection in research.

There are also competency sets developed for particular types of public health professionals including public health leaders and administrators, and public health professionals in clinical services evaluating individuals and families, in epidemiology and data management, in population-based health education, in laboratory sciences, and professionals in environmental health.

Few, if any, public health education programs have developed comprehensive curricula in genomics. Genomics is not only new, but also changing as rapidly as any area of bioscience. This combination presents a particularly daunting challenge to designing curricula. Schools and programs need to integrate a largely new content area while, at the same time, recognizing that what is currently known, even at the cutting-edge frontiers of that content area will be woefully out of date and/or incorrect early in their students' professional lives. Thus, public health curricula in genomics may need to focus on creating a framework of appreciation for the importance of genomics and a basic understanding of the topic.

It has long been widely agreed in the field of genomics that its ethical, legal, and social implications (ELSI) are important for society at large and, particularly so, for health professionals. In educating students about genetics and genomics, programs and schools of public health have a responsibility to consider these issues. Some of these ELSI issues are included in each of the two organizations' sets of competencies cited above. Undoubtedly new issues that we cannot yet foresee will arise in this area during the professional lives of today's students. Thus, it is important that schools of public health constantly update their curricula in all areas of genomics, including the ELSI issues.

Ethical, legal, and social issues are important to many areas in the education of students of public health, including genomics. Therefore, it is important that consideration of these issues not be an afterthought or an ancillary part of education in genomics. The curriculum needs to include ELSI issues as a basic, essential component of its genomics instruction; indeed, no school of public health can be thought to teach genomics effectively or appropriately if its curriculum fails to do so. Similarly, faculty responsible for this area of the curriculum must have real expertise in the subject area.

Advances in genomics hold great promise for future improvements in health. However it is not only the future of genomics that warrants the attention of public health education. Because few in the current public health workforce have the level of understanding of genomics that is required today, major continuing education efforts must be undertaken to ready practicing public heath professionals to use genomics effectively. Public health education programs and schools must provide their students with a framework for understanding the importance of genomics to public health and with the ability to apply genomics to basic public health sciences.

COMMUNICATION

The role of public health in the daily lives of U.S. citizens has become increasingly prominent at the same time that evidence of gaps in the training of public health professionals has emerged. A critical gap is the need for understanding and skills-based performance and practice in communication. The body of knowledge associated with communication has evolved to the extent that evidence-based research affords a solid core to guide public health professionals' training in this domain. Reflecting this fact, for the first time since its adoption in 1979, the Healthy People framework for providing a national prevention agenda included a chapter on Health Communication in the 2010 objectives. In this chapter health communication is defined as

> the art and technique of informing, influencing, and motivating individual, institutional, and public audiences about important health issues. The scope of health communication includes disease prevention, health promotion, health care policy, and the business of health care as well as enhancement of the quality of life and health of individuals within the community (U.S. DHHS, 2000).

As emphasized within an ecological model, public health professionals interact with groups representing all the foci addressed in the 2010 definition of health communication. An examination of past successes and failures in public health emphasizes this reality. Whether working with communities, interacting with members of the lay public from different cultural backgrounds, or making the case for public health to Congress, communication forms the foundation on which these efforts are built. Public health professionals depend upon being perceived as credible, with the creation and maintenance of images of trustworthiness and expertise occurring more often by intention than accident and dependent upon effective communication.

Public Health Communication Defined

As a form of health communication, public health communication involves a translation process that begins with the basic science of what is known about a health topic. From the science, public health professionals derive messages about attitudes and behaviors the public should adopt, together with policies that organizations and government should enact to support population health. Public health professionals often communicate within a learning model approach in which practices are based on the formation of attitudes that are derived from knowledge and contribute to the ability to make informed choices about their health (Valente et al., 1998). Public health professionals sell products, services, and/or points of view, making strategic communication in the form of social marketing common (Cirksena and Flora, 1995). The attainment of communication goals associated with social marketing depends upon audience analysis to segment "publics" and guides the design of relevant messages. Social marketers focus on the *product* as an idea, behavior, or item that they want to be accepted, evaluating the *price* in terms of costs associated with adoption, including economic but also social and psychological barriers. *Promotion* of the product occurs with these costs in mind, together with attention to placing the promotion where a particular audience will gain access to it at an appropriate time (Parrott et al., 1998a). Public health professionals who want the public to be aware of food safety inspections, for example, may strive to "place" these ratings at the entrance of restaurants.

A common term used in the process of translating science to public health communication is "risk." Risk communication addresses a negative event or hazard that threatens the public's safety, with communication about that hazard focusing on the probability of its occurrence multiplied by its magnitude, weighed together with consideration of less quantifiable factors such as social values (Covello, 1992). Public health professionals may intend to communicate particular meanings when using the term "risk" in their messages, but policy making and public audiences who receive the messages interpret them based on their own experiences, including cultural, social, and personal frameworks (Carrese and Rhodes, 1995; Glasgow et al., 1999). Beliefs that a risk is voluntary, under one's own control, has clear benefits, is fairly distributed, and/or occurs naturally contribute to acceptance of risk as compared to beliefs that a risk is imposed, is controlled by others, has little benefit, is unfairly distributed, or is manmade (Fischhoff, 1999).

Public health professionals who apply this knowledge to communication with different audiences would consider that a critical component of assessing the "price" associated with adopting a "product" is analysis of costs versus benefits (Fishbein and Ajzen, 1975) and recognize that humans usually resist communication that arouses feelings that freedoms are being violated (Brehm, 1966; Engs and Hanson, 1989). These and other frameworks may be applied to increase the effectiveness of public health communication.

Strategies to Facilitate Public Health Communication

Public health professionals should plan risk communication to include strategies for coping with risk rather than just information about risk. Communicating these guidelines together with information about a risk will enable the public to have a sense of confidence and control, contributing to perceived self-efficacy in abilities and skills to adapt to a situation (Bandura, 1986). When communicating about health, prescriptions frequently become injunctions to avoid behaviors that relate to individual occupations, recreational pursuits, and cultural backgrounds. *Communication science may be summarized to predict that individuals will behave in ways that promote their health and well being more often when they are asked to adapt to rather than avoid health risks.* Behavior adaptation is more likely when individuals:

- have access to the information, products, and services associated with adapting to health risk;
- hold accurate procedural knowledge about strategies to adapt to risk;
- perceive themselves to have such knowledge;
- perceive those in their personal networks as expecting them to adapt to the risk; and
- make a public commitment to adapt to risk (Parrott et al., 1998b).

Public health communication sometimes includes statistics, at other times depends upon personal narratives, and often combines the two, communicating through the use of multiple channels, including varied forms of media such as television and radio, but also in combination with interpersonal channels such as health educators and/or public health nurses. Use of multiple channels has been found to be more effective in changing behavior than reliance on a single modality (Schooler et al., 1998), as long as the message remains consistent.

Communication about health exists in environments cluttered with inconsistent messages and unable to support many prescribed practices. Individuals must cope with public health recommendations to exercise in ecological environments where air quality does not support the practice, drink water when water quality has been reported to be poor, and follow a host of other messages that often can be attributed to public health professionals (Parrott et al., 2002). Conflicting health information causes perceptions that, regardless of what we do, we will be unable to control our future health (Wortman and Brehm, 1975). Public health professionals want to avoid such perceptions. Thus, in using multiple channels, public health professionals should be trained to recognize conflicting messages that may occur as a result of different values associated with reporting the news versus informing the public about health.

News depends on controversy and magnitude to make a story more personally relevant (Bell, 1991). These values sometimes conflict with efforts to avoid distorting public health information and contribute to the general public's perceptions that private information will be made public as a result of interaction with the public health system.

Barriers to Overcome in Public Health Communication

The public's cooperation with public health goals includes disclosing personal information in medical and public health settings, contributing to the collection of data for disease registries, allocating resources to health and health care needs, and recognizing gaps in policy and health law. A population perspective to communicating about health may be a barrier at the level of the individual who must disclose personal information to promote the public's health. Public health professionals communicate with many different audiences, which may cause concern about the confidentiality associated with personal information and violations of privacy.

If members of the public are uncertain about how disclosing personal information may affect health insurance coverage, personal relationships, and/or their own self concept, they may avoid participating in public health activities perceived to threaten these areas, with computerization of health information increasing such avoidance (Brown and Levinson, 1978; Parrott et al., 2001). People living with AIDS and cancer survivors, as well as African Americans living with the legacy of Tuskeegee illustrate direct experience with such concerns. Moreover, members of the lay public who live in rural areas where public health agencies often seek to fill the gap in access to information, products, and services exhibit extended social interconnectedness. These relationships have an impact on confidentiality and require extra vigilance in efforts to safeguard information and to communicate how confidentiality will be maintained (Ullom-Muinich and Kallail, 1993).

Public health professionals may increase individual confidence in these efforts by limiting the number of questions asked, evaluating the content of information requests, restricting access to individual information, and securing adequate space to accommodate individuals so that they will not be overheard (Parrott, 1995), which are intentional efforts associated with maintaining public health professionals' credibility.

To balance the goals of population health with the rights and concerns of individual citizens, public health communication should be conducted within a framework associated with communication that does not raise expectations that cannot be met (Guttman, 1997). In these efforts, public health professionals must balance knowledge of strategies to involve audiences with efforts to avoid manipulating information so that lay audiences do what public health professionals want them to do. Public health communication should contribute to the adoption of policies and regulations that safeguard public health, while respecting individual rights to privacy. Moreover, public health professionals must acknowledge that different groups vary in the access they have to the personal and societal resources needed for them to be informed about public health or act on public health promotion recommendations. Thus, without careful efforts to conceptualize and assess the environment, public health communication may widen gaps between knowledge and behavior.

Public Health Communication Competence

Public health professionals require different communication skills to interact with various publics, including co-workers, elected officials and policymakers, health care providers, media, and lay citizens, all comprising the public health professionals' sphere of influence. At a macro level, public health professionals should be able to state the case for public health programs and activities, which often requires knowledge of the history of public health promotion and research efforts associated with a topic, an audience, and one's own agency and area. Cross-cutting skills associated with public health communication include the ability to conduct audience analysis to assess perceptions associated with "risk" (voluntary, control, distribution equity, natural) and audience perspectives of costs versus benefits of health-promoting behaviors and policies. This requires training in traditional and innovative formative evaluation strategies to uncover individual, community, and societal models associated with health and health care issues, and implicit costs versus benefits of healthy and unhealthy habits. Public health professionals also need skills to assess what and how information is being collected from the public, keeping these to a minimum to enhance disclosure.

Public health professionals work with and respond to communities to monitor the public's health. Communities exist in a social environment that includes the health knowledge, attitudes, and practices of families, friends, co-workers, and others in the social network as they relate to a designated campaign topic. Training is needed to assess supportive as compared to unsupportive characteristics of the existing environments associated with public health goals. Access to information, products, and services associated with public health action and promotion is necessary but not sufficient to support population health. Social processes contribute to definitions of health within a group and should be assessed in terms of whether personal and/or social responsibility is compatible with group values. The message environment may include inconsistent guidelines for treatment and prevention that need to be addressed. National, social, and political agendas and biases direct what is and is not communicated to the public about health. Public health professionals' training should support their skills in identifying these situations.

Public health professionals will work with and respond to the news in efforts to make policy and evolve public health strategies. Media advocacy acknowledges this relationship and strives to strategically plan for and use news to educate and involve community members with important issues (Wallack and Dorfman, 2001). Public health communication requires skills to use mass media strategically in combination with community organizing to advance public health policies through media advocacy, targeting policymakers, organizations, and/or legislative bodies. Public health professionals should be able to frame public health problems as social inequities to derive policy solutions, as well as apply news values and advertising principles to design stories about these public health issues for media outlets. Public health professionals should also be able to identify people, groups, and/or organizations that have the authority, power, and influence to create and change policy, and work with them to increase exposure and reach of messages. This often requires skills in working effectively with media gatekeepers to build media partnerships and access strategies, and in designing and conducting media evaluation research.

Finally, public health professionals' communication illustrates a longstanding ethical dilemma between utility and justice, and training should be examined with such issues in the forefront, emphasizing the application of ethical principles to communication about health and health information. Public health professionals should be able to evaluate strategic communication for evidence that information is being distorted to achieve public health aims. They should also look for unintended outcomes that may occur as a result of communication. Such unintended outcomes include labeling some members of the public, depriving individuals of affordable pleasures or important resources (e.g., time), and/or a focus on personal responsibility when societal conditions cause the public health threat.

Public health professionals' job expectations will be more readily met through training and education in communication. Such training should emphasize the role of individual level theories in explaining information seeking and processing as well as individual judgments and decision-making, individual and societal level theories focusing on the interrelationships between individuals and groups or media and gatekeeping processes, and societal level theories relating to social, political, and economic theories of health. Derived from these theories are guidelines for suggesting how public health professionals may attain skills for practice relating to collecting and interpreting formative data at the individual level; working with diverse audiences and groups, including policymakers and opinion leaders at the individual and societal levels; reframing issues as societal rather than individual; and analyzing and formulating public policy (Maibach et al., 1994).

CULTURAL COMPETENCE

Globalization, changing demographics, and disparities in health care have brought renewed attention to cultural competence skills and information in public health education and training. The term cultural competence has been so heavily overworked that it is often perceived and responded to as an empty cliché or ideology (Vega and Lopez, 2001). How is it possible to address the cultural variety inherent in the social world and to incorporate the most essential information within public health education? Where are the incentives to do so? These are difficult questions, and time will be required to develop or create adequate responses to them. Scientists do not resist investigation of the human genome because it represents too much variety; the same scientific logic works equally well for sorting and classifying information about culture, ethnicity, and race. Culture has many meanings and expressions; however the role of public health practitioners is to determine which sociocultural aspects are most relevant to their mission.

Cultural competence in public health is a systematic process. Its purpose is to change public health practice by effective education and training of public health students and practitioners. Cultural *sensitivity*, on the other hand, is rooted in developing attitudes of respect and appreciation for individual and cultural difference, and forms a foundation and rationale for cultural competence. Cultural competence is based on an empirically derived body of knowledge that is translated and integrated into the curricula and an established stock of knowledge imparted in programs and schools of public health. This process is accomplished by translating knowledge into skill sets that are continuously reviewed, refined, and disseminated. Cultural competency should be defined through operational criteria. These cultural competence criteria can be infused into public health organizations at all levels, staff development, reward structures, community assessments, developing community outreach or stakeholder involvement, planning community programs, distribution of human resources, and system change. Similar practice skills and criteria pertain to community research and evaluation because they affect selection of topics, design of research, development and selection of measures, data analyses, and interpretation of findings.

The goal in cultural competence education is to increase public health professionals' cultural awareness, knowledge of self and others, communication skills, attitudes, and behaviors. Part of this process is confronting stereotypes, because many students entering public health have minimal experience with ethnic minorities. This is accomplished by a systematic exposure to a knowledge base that, combined with practice methods, provides an additional dimension to public health education. The knowledge base includes specificity about inter-ethnic and intra-ethnic health indices, sociocultural aspects of health and help seeking, assessment techniques adapted to community cultural diversity, improving communication of health prevention and promotion, and medical care information, cultural translation and mobilization strategies for communities and their institutions, and methodologies to improve the delivery of public health interventions and to evaluate their effectiveness (Lee, 1988; Gold, 1992; Mo, 1992; Alcalay et al., 1993; Vega and VanOss-Marin, 1997; House and Williams, 2000; Kaplan et al., 2000; Schulz et al., 2001).

The need for cross-cultural sensitivity becomes apparent when placed in a global context. Other societies, such as Chinese, South Indian, and African societies have rich traditions in the medical arts that are centuries old and based on an epistemology that is distinct from western thought and action. Cross-cultural sensitivity is no less important for public health within the United States. There are now in excess of 80 million people in the United States in the four groups customarily categorized as "minorities": African Americans, Hispanics, American Indians, and Asians and Pacific Islanders (U.S. Census, 2001). There are many other people, perhaps less visible, whose cultural background or sexual orientation places them outside the cultural mainstream.

Definitive reviews have appeared from authoritative sources highlighting disparities in health status, barriers to services, and lower quality of medical care received by minorities. The Office of Minority Health (U.S. DHHS, 2002b) issued a report, *Teaching Cultural Competence in Health Care*, where current concepts, policies and practices were reviewed. This report identifies several recommended cultural competence guidelines and standards issued by professional groups such as the American Psychological Association (APA), the American Medical Association (AMA), the National Association of Social Workers (NASW), the American Public Health Association (APHA), and minority medical associations. The Institute of Medicine (IOM) (2002) released a report that carefully describes and documents how disparities are pervasive and manifested in the organization and delivery of medical care, resulting in consistently inferior health status and treatment outcomes for minorities. Among the most important factors cited in both reports are low health care access, poverty, poor patient communication (including cultural conflicts and language problems), racism, and discrimination. Although the public health mission is not focused primarily on medical care, there is ample experiential and empirical evidence that these same key factors should be addressed in programs and schools of public health through research, comprehensive curricular integration, and practice.

The need to contour public health according to the cultural ways of different groups is an important theme in the public health literature. For instance, substance abuse prevention practitioners working in cross-cultural settings are advised to be inclusive of those who have a stake in the program if resistance is to be minimized (Orlandi, 1992; Scott, 1990); to use multiple methods that may emphasize oral traditions versus written and experimental protocols (Airhihenbuwa, 1995); to take into account factors that are not only behavioral, but also contextual (Braithwaite and Taylor, 1992); and to learn how to gain access and trust in forging cross-cultural relationships by being aware of and sensitive to cultural nuances in interacting with others (Airhihenbuwa, 1995). These elements are shared by writers concerned with communities that are African American (Grace, 1992), Hispanic (Casas, 1992), American Indian (Beauvais and Trimble, 1992), and Asian/Pacific Islander (Yen, 1992). Lack of cultural competence in domestic practice is one of the factors that guides the objectives in *Healthy People 2010* (U.S. DHHS, 2000). Educators, researchers, and practitioners must intensify their efforts to ensure that public health students are properly prepared to address the needs of these populations.

The Council on Linkages Between Academia and Public Health Practice has developed eight competency domains for public health professionals, one of which is cultural competency. The committee believes that this core competency as explicated by the council is important and forms a focus for education of culturally competent public health professionals. Ultimately, all areas of public health instruction are encompassed by cultural competence to a greater or lesser degree. The exploration of cultural competence improves core skills including attention to cultural-linguistic nuance in health screening, improving the ability of public health professionals to pose and answer research questions, redesigning interventions to fit ethnic community environments, and evaluating health policy issues. Improving screening for cancer, diabetes, and heart disease, increasing exercise regularity, reducing toxic exposures, stopping tobacco use, reducing HIV risk, and helping individuals make informed decisions about health care providers are examples of typical public health projects improved by cultural competence. Cultural competence includes supplying students with better interpersonal communication tools for entering multi-ethnic communities to conduct research and interventions. There are now many research articles, books, and Web sites available that offer information and additional resources to provide a concrete foundation for commencing cultural competence instruction in programs and schools of public health. The next step is to integrate this information where it is needed across the curricula and to continue refining the knowledge base and pedagogy of cultural competence.

Cultural and ethnic awareness must also be increased in public health research. There has been relatively slow progress in including ethnic minorities in public health research and intervention trials. In recent years federal requirements at the National Institutes of Health (NIH) have made the inclusion of ethnic minorities nearly compulsory in research. However, these requirements pertain primarily to participation of human subjects in research. There are no guidelines about researcher responsibility or ethical practices when research is conducted in minority communities. In addition criteria have not been established for adequacy of research designs that increase the likelihood of high quality research results with external validity for minority populations. Minority communities often are suspicious of, or even hostile to, public health researchers because they have seen little benefit or improved conditions within their own communities from previous research.

Padilla and Medina (1996) assert that cultural sensitivity should span the entire research study process, including the adaptation, translation, and administration of measures, along with the analysis, scoring, and interpretation of results. Without such cultural adaptations, biases may occur that can lead to misinterpretation of a program's results (Keitel et al., 1996). To reduce culturally induced bias, Suzuki et al. (1996) offer the following suggestions: develop alternative measures and procedures for diverse populations, understand the norms of ethnic groups to which evaluations are applied, increase collaboration with bilingual and bicultural professionals in developing evaluations, increase racial and ethnic community involvement in the assessment process, and consult the literature and research available regarding multicultural assessment procedures.

Orlandi conceptualized what he terms an "expert linkage approach," in which public health experts are brought together with members of a cultural group and each is accorded equal significance in the collaboration. The approach is similar to that identified in the section on community-based participatory practices; therefore, the skills required are also similar. In particular, cross-cultural competence requires the public health professional to combine the perspective of a group that is the focus of study or practice with the science that informs public health research and practice. To do so means that professional training should include courses in cross-cultural understanding that are influenced by anthropology and other similar disciplines. Additionally, training in methodology should be multioperational, thus exposing the learner to a broad array of methods that take into account cultures in which oral (and other non-Western) traditions predominate. Training should focus on ways in which methods can be adapted in partnership with cross-cultural groups and still retain scientific validity.

Cultural competence skills and knowledge are applicable to dual priorities in public health education, global health, and U.S. ethnic minority health. There is substantial overlap in the cross-cultural and linguistic challenges each area presents for improving public health education. Thus, it is logical and parsimonious for programs and schools of public health to disseminate cultural competence skills that are applicable in a transnational context, bearing in mind the inescapable truth that local public health practice requires local knowledge—including awareness of the cultural world, its heterogeneity, resources, and conflicts.

Several schools of public health have strong international health programs that already emphasize the importance of cross-cultural understanding and the adaptation of practices for working outside of the United States. They may serve as models that may be more widely adopted and applied to both international and domestic public health.

A fundamental challenge in achieving cultural competency in public health education and research is the need to increase the number of students and faculty from under-represented minority groups. In some instances these groups represent a cultural continuum extending from nations of origin in Latin America, Asia, Africa, the Caribbean, and Europe, to new communities of resettlement in the United States. The volume of students from many of these ethnic groups in public health education is inadequate, especially blacks and Latinos, who comprise nearly 90 percent of the total U.S. minority population.

Although data are scarce, a recent unpublished inquiry conducted by faculty of Columbia University found that about 40 percent ($n = 12$) of the 29 respondent schools of public health offered no specific courses on minority health in 2001 (Personal Communication, M. Aguirre-Molina, Columbia University, June 15, 2002). A total of 34 courses were offered among the remaining 17 schools, and of these, 29 were general survey (overview) courses. Only 10 schools offered 2 or more courses on health issues of minorities. This brief profile suggests that with few exceptions, U.S. schools of public health are poorly positioned to adequately motivate or prepare students for addressing disparities in health among minority populations.

The absence of undergraduate degree programs in public health at many schools delays the potential exposure of minority candidates, thus decreasing the number of recruits available for graduate training directly from undergraduate schools. Mentoring programs in the sciences have been developed at the NIH for high school students from minority backgrounds to better equip them to compete academically at the university level, thus increasing their survival rates for advanced career preparation in the sciences. However, most of these programs are limited to the biological sciences. The minority pipelines at the secondary school and community college levels are poorly developed for public health. Even high school magnet programs in the health sciences tend to focus on classic career tracks, such as nursing and medicine. Public health has not established sufficient visibility in this arena and has received little federal support or leadership to do so. This must change.

Programs and schools of public health must demonstrate leadership and creativity in developing outreach programs in their local areas. They could sponsor courses in public health and help high schools implement their own courses by providing technical assistance. One such program has been developed by the University of California at Los Angeles School of Public Health. This program offers an introductory public health course at a local community college for both high school and community college students. The objective is to expose students to the opportunities available for positively improving their communities through a career in public health. Special programs on minority health accompanied by outreach to minority communities, secondary schools, and community colleges could also be created.

A related issue is the wholly inadequate supply of minority faculty. This is compounded by a dearth of tenured faculty that have direct experience with public health practice in minority communities. Some faculty may even be attitudinally resistant or substantively unprepared to address the renovation of curricula to achieve greater cultural competence among their students. Programs and schools must be willing to engage in reform and leadership development and to examine mechanisms for attracting, training, and retaining faculty from minority backgrounds.

The "pipeline" issue requires attention and action. A comprehensive approach is needed to identify, encourage, and support a greater diversity of students in schools and programs of public health, and to help those students complete their graduate degrees at the masters and doctoral levels. Greater attention should be given to undergraduate courses in public health that specifically address minority health issues and to developing outreach efforts to minority organizations to garner their assistance in reaching minority students. Programs could be established to partially or wholly support education to earn a master of public health (M.P.H.) degree for qualified minority scholars with doctorates in needed fields such as the social and behavioral sciences of psychology, sociology, demography, anthropology, etc.

The practice of public health requires culturally competent public health professionals who know how to effectively communicate public health messages to an increasingly diverse population. These messages must be based on high quality information, obtained in a timely fashion, and shared in a manner that respects the values, opinions, beliefs, and practices of the communities with which public health interacts. In an era of expanded awareness of health disparities and an emphasis on prevention, do we have the requisite knowledge to reach ethnic minority communities and create awareness of specific health threats and reduce population risk? Will the enriched public health infrastructure adequately incorporate the needs of ethnic and cultural minorities? These are long-range challenges. Some progress has been made, but an active use of technological capability is needed to identify and rapidly disseminate cultural competency information and to integrate it into the core competency curricula. The importance of supervised practical experience to the mastering of cultural competency cannot be overstated. This may require some public health faculty to augment their own personal experience in minority communities in order to provide improved student field supervision and classroom instruction.

Cultural competency must emerge from the category of "necessary nuisance" that it too often occupies, which both isolates and trivializes its role. Cultural competency should be supported as an essential element in teaching, research, and practice.

COMMUNITY-BASED PARTICIPATORY RESEARCH

Public health research has contributed greatly to improvements in population- and individual-level health. Basic research, conducted for the purpose of advancing our knowledge, has helped us learn about such things as the basic biology of infectious agents (e.g., viruses and bacteria) and the biochemical and molecular mechanisms by which specific environmental factors cause or contribute to chronic diseases. Applied or translational research, designed to use the results of other research to solve real world problems, helps us understand, for example, how antibiotic resistance develops in certain types of organisms, so that the most effective treatments can be used. Evaluative research can be used to help us analyze the impact of welfare reform on the health of immigrant children or the effectiveness of high blood pressure prevention programs. Descriptive research that attempts to discover facts or describe reality provides us with hypothesis-generating studies, epidemiological studies, observational studies, and surveys. A prime example of this type of study is the original Framingham study that led to identification of risk factors for cardiovascular disease in middle-aged adults. All of these types of research are crucial to the field of public health and continue to be necessary components of the public health research portfolio.

Additionally, given the demographic transformations in the United States, there is increasing need to incorporate lessons learned about community engagement, and the complex nature of interventions into community-based research. Community-based research is an overarching concept of collaborative research that encompasses many different types of studies, for example, applied, descriptive, and evaluative. Green and Mercer (2001) define participatory research as "an approach that entails involving all potential users of the research and other stakeholders in the formulation as well as the application of the research." According to Green and Mercer, maximum participation occurs when the stakeholders remain active throughout the study—posing the research question, engaging in the selection and application of methods, and applying the findings. Minimum participation requires involvement in question formulation, interpretation, and application of findings. To Green and Mercer, the focus on participation separates community research from basic and applied research, with basic research involving only the researcher, and applied involving the research and practitioners.

Israel and colleagues (2001) define community-based participatory research (CBPR) as "a partnership approach to research that equitably involves community members, organizational representatives, and researchers in all aspects of the research process." Whereas Green and Mercer focus on the participatory quality of the research, Israel and colleagues anchor the approach in geographically defined communities. Thus, CBPR and the training that it requires is most linked to practice in geographically-determined community settings. The NIH National Institute of Environmental Health Sciences defines community-based participatory research as a methodology that promotes active community involvement in the processes that shape research and intervention strategies, as well as in the conduct of research studies (NIH, 2002).

A Rationale for CBPR and Practice

Green and Mercer (2001) observe that communities often find that they participate in research that has limited applicability and is insensitive to the community in the process. Lack of access to and cooperation from community groups are common ramifications of poor relationships with communities. The breach in relationships also is discussed in the IOM reports on the future of public health (1988) and linkages between research and practice (1997). It is further recognized by investigators who have wrestled with the complexities of community research and who have helped reshape public health programming in community settings over the past 25 years. For instance, in considering the mixed record in protecting the integrity of research subjects, Strauss et al. (2001) propose that community advisory boards be established to minimize the possibility of ethical violations of research participants' rights. The authors define the functions required of investigators in the research process, including the following:

- maximize the participants' ability to make informed decisions;
- assure that participation is voluntary;
- reveal openly all ramifications of the research; and
- accommodate community concerns about design or conduct of the research.

In addition to the ethical considerations that incorporate active oversight by community groups, the complex nature of the interventions underscores the importance of CBPR approaches. Of particular note are the 10 year community trials in the late 1970s and early 1980s, funded by the National Heart, Lung and Blood Institute (NHLBI), and directed at cardiovascular risk reduction (Farquhar et al., 1985; Elder et al., 1986; Jacobs et al., 1986; Mittelmark et al., 1993). Each implemented numerous community activities that included risk factor screening, general and specific media messages, work site physical activity, menu labeling at restaurants, grocery labeling, school programs, work with health practitioners, community-wide contests, community task forces, and speakers bureaus, as well as others (Jacobs et al., 1986).

The lessons learned about community engagement from these complex community trials were reinforced during the last decade by the emergence of social ecology principles for informing public health interventions (Shinn, 1996; Green and Kreuter, 1999). Social ecology is the application of multiple and linked intervention strategies across multiple social levels—the individual, family, social network, service organizations, community groups, and policy bodies (Goodman, 2000a; McLeroy et al., 1988). Stokols and colleagues (1996) suggest that research and practice based on comprehensive ecological formulations are needed in community health because limited intervention programs produce high relapse and attrition rates.

Empirical evidence is accumulating that suggests that CBPR approaches are consequential in producing important outcomes. As discussed earlier, in CBPR the community is a full partner in identifying the research questions to be addressed. These research questions are not developed or structured in the same manner as those posed by the quantitative researcher nor are they necessarily hypothesis driven, and they are not determined a priori and out of context from the communities in which the solutions arise. The National Institute of Environmental Health Sciences (NIEHS) funded a community-based participatory research project in Oregon aimed at reducing pesticide exposures in families. Participants included migrant farm workers, community representatives, analytical chemists, epidemiologists, exposure assessment scientists, investigators skilled in qualitative research methods, and neurobehavioral scientists. According to NIEHS, "the blend of each of these areas of expertise allows for the generation of information to the community (e.g., workshops, training videos) and scientific information on the pesticide exposures of farm workers and their families and the effects of exposures on human health. The community benefits from the increased knowledge of the nature and extent of pesticide exposures in their work and home environments while the basic and applied scientist gains an increased sensitivity of community priorities and the need for culturally appropriate research methods and communication (www.niehs.nih.gov/translat/cbr-final.pdf). Further examples of successful CBPR projects can be found in the NIEHS report entitled *Successful Models of Community-Based Participatory Research* at (www.niehs.nih.gov/translat/cbr-final.pdf).

The CBPR approach has developed in response to the lack of success of other approaches that excluded the community from the research process (Green and Mercer, 2001). As with other evolving approaches (e.g., genomics, an important area for research that we support in the present report), much of the evidence base is emergent. Currently, CBPR approaches are receiving a great deal of attention from the public health community. CDC recently funded 25 community-based research projects founded on CBPR principles (Personal Communication, L. Green, Centers for Disease Control and Prevention, September 13, 2002), and the June 2002 issue of *Health Education & Behavior*, the most widely cited journal in the Health Education field, devoted an entire special issue to the topic (Schulz et al., 2002).

In short, the underlying rationale for CBPR and practice entails increased sensitivity to a community's rightful place as a partner in research and practice. Furthermore, practical considerations dictate that community cooperation is predicated on processes that are participatory. Lastly, complex, interventions require communities to work in partnership with researchers and providers. Without comprehensive community approaches, pockets of prevalence may not be addressed effectively.

CBPR and Other Approaches

Community Research and Practice

Israel et al. (2001) draw a distinction between CBPR as "community-based" and other approaches as "community-placed." The 1997 IOM report on linkages between research and practice draws a similar distinction for research projects, noting three levels:

1) current proactive practice of academically driven research initiatives,

2) a more reactive practice for designing research in response to the needs and input of community agencies,

3) the development of interactive practices that involve both academic researchers and the community as equal partners in all phases of a research project.

The first level of research typically involves the researcher as the sole inquirer (Green and Mercer's definition of *basic research*). The second level involves community concerns with academicians defining the methods of inquiry and the range of answers (Green and Mercer's definition of *applied research*). The third type enjoins community representatives and academicians in collective exploration (Green's and Mercer's definition of *participatory research*). Three levels of practice that are analogous to the research levels include:

1) community programs that often have minimum input from community organizations and/or community members (public health clinics may be one such example),

2) collaborative models in which community organizations and members join programs with predetermined practices (WIC [the Women, Infants, and Children program] may be one such example),

3) efforts that involve joint definitions of processes and outcomes (REACH [Racial and Ethnic Approach to Community Health] may be one such example).

Proponents of CBPR and practice view them as distinct paradigmatically from levels 1 and 2, whereas the 1997 IOM report views the three types as a continuum along which research may evolve.

Social Determinants of Health

Research into social determinants of health (SDOH) is another area that has implications for community engagement and that can be distinguished from CBPR. SDOH has its foundations in social epidemiology, particularly that aspect which focuses on social inequalities in contributing to disease and disability (Berkman and Kawachi, 2000). A concentration on social inequalities incorporates the study of social determinants of health (SDOH), or factors that contribute to "how society shapes the health of people" (Berkman and Kawachi, 2000). The SDOH perspective shares many characteristics with social ecology principles in that both take a population perspective, highlight social context in understanding individual behavior, and operate on multiple social levels.

SDOH may be distinguished from social protective factors (SPF), or conditions that can mitigate social ills. For instance, Krieger (2000) enumerates research studies on the effects of discrimination on a range of health outcomes, including blood pressure, hypertension, cigarette smoking, depression, and other forms of psychological distress. Thus, discrimination as a social determinant is linked empirically to health outcomes. The question remains, what can public health offer in the face of pernicious social determinants like discrimination, poverty, and job dislocation? One practical response is to study other SPF that may have salutary effects on a community's health.

Community capacity is one example of a cluster of SPF that do not necessarily reduce the presence of negative determinants like discrimination, but may bolster proactive community responses in the face of such determinants. Currently, CDC funds several special interest projects to understand how community capacity may improve community health outcomes. Measures for capacity, social capital, and SPF are in development. Preliminary findings indicate that communities that are most successful in producing desired community health and social outcomes tend to have important capacities in leadership, a strong set of values and principles, organizing abilities, and strategic community actions. Although these findings remain preliminary, they reinforce the prominent role that community-based participatory research and practice should be accorded in public health. SDOH and SPF are mutually supportive approaches, with the former focusing on the social context that produces social disparities, disease, and disability (sometimes referred to as "downstream" approaches), and SPF focusing on community-based interventions that may augur resistance to harmful social conditions (sometimes referred to as "upstream" approaches).

Skills Training in CBPR and Practice

Israel and colleagues (2001) characterize CBPR as incorporating several operating principles including the following:

- the central place that communities are accorded as units of identity and as co-equals in research;
- a process that is not perceived by community constituents as university-dominated or elitist;
- the emphasis on long-term commitment by all partners;
- the emphasis on co-learning so that the process flows back and forth;
- the use of exercises that stimulate collective visioning among all partners;
- the incorporation of social ecology approaches as departures for

research and practice;
   • the use of innovative problem-solving approaches;
   • the use of multiple methods of data collection to produce a rich and textured picture of partnership functioning and the outcomes that will result.

Israel and colleagues also suggest that challenges in implementing CBPR include the following:

   • the time and effort required to build trust and true partnering;
   • the difficulties in developing a common purpose;
   • the challenges of working with partners from diverse backgrounds and experiences;
   • the practical constraints that compromise CBPR principles in practice;
   • the difficulties in reaching balance and equity in the distribution of resources and other benefits.

The principles and challenges suggest the skills necessary to conduct CBPR and practice. For many researchers and practitioners, the development of new skills or the modification of existing skills will be required, including the ability to collaborate and share control in decision making and action regarding program design, implementation, and evaluation; the non-trivial use of community resources, skills, and relationships; and the cultivation of new capacities and partnerships among organizations and individuals (Paxman et al., 2000). Several programs at schools of public health teach skills in CBPR (e.g., University of Michigan). The curricula from these programs may provide guidance for establishing additional training requirements.

Skills that foster collaborative control in decision making and action

Researchers engaged in CBPR are program stakeholders, collaborators, and builders of capacity for the community interventions. They provide continuous feedback during each stage of a community program's development. To reach the stage at which the researchers (or practitioners) can work collaboratively with community groups, they must learn skills to gain entrée into the community and to foster cooperation and trust among various community groups. They must have competencies in team building, group process, negotiation, developing consensus, teaching, interpersonal communication, and the acquisition of political acumen. Programs and schools of public health have at least three important roles that they can take in training researchers and practitioners to use community-based participatory approaches. First, course work on community engagement concepts should be integrated into the M.P.H.

curriculum. Topics to include involve community theory, development strategies, promising interventions, group development techniques, community diagnosis, and capacity assessments. Secondly, the practicum or capstone experience should incorporate community-based experience. In many instances, students receive no academic credit for this requirement, and little faculty time is devoted to group discussions or debriefing sessions with students regarding community practice. The practicum or capstone experience may be used more fully to train in community-based approaches. Third, faculty should be encouraged to include students on funded community-based research enterprises. Research clusters of faculty and students that work on ongoing community projects can form academic "incubators" for growing mature community researchers and practitioners.

Technical competencies—research and evaluation

Many facets of community-based research and evaluation are unique. For instance, in CBPR the researcher provides continuous feedback to the community. In classical research approaches, such incursions by the researcher are considered to be threats to internal validity because the researcher influences the intervention. In research that is participatory, the investigator learns to develop methods for assuring internal validity that may deviate from classical approaches (Goodman, 2000b). Moreover, the movement towards multiple, complex, and community-based interventions has implications for redefining the types of skills required to research and practice community public health approaches. Flay (1986) focused on the impediments in implementing complex community programs, including reaching the planned targets at the correct time with adequate intensity and desired effects. Altman (1986) sought methods for disaggregating program components to understand the multiple causal mechanisms within complex community interventions.

Research, development, and assessment of community programs are difficult because they are necessarily different in different communities, need to be flexible and responsive to changing local needs and conditions, have broad and multiple goals, take many years to produce major outcomes, and require multiple data collection and analysis methods extended over long periods of time (Goodman, 2000b). Programs and schools of public health should have a central role in training researchers and practitioners to research, implement, and evaluate complex community interventions. The implications for programs and schools of public health concerning training for CBPR and practice are that multiple methods are important given the complexities of community health factors. The researcher, evaluator, and practitioner should be trained to tailor strategies to the specific questions and concerns of a community project.

In developing the widest array of possible strategies, the public health profession requires training in both quantitative and qualitative approaches. Quantitative approaches typically use statistical techniques to judge whether program recipients benefit from the program in contrast to controls or comparisons. Qualitative approaches seldom use randomization and often do not have comparison groups; rather they focus on the program itself and use detailed observations of activities and events, interviews with program stakeholders, and reviews of program documents to judge program results. Moreover, new approaches should be incorporated as they develop. For instance, recent advances in geographic information systems (GIS) technology allows for increased availability and interpretation of geographic or location-based information (Richards et al., 1999).

Beyond the learning techniques, part of student training requires adeptness at community consultation as the basis for making adaptations in research, evaluation, and practice designs so that they hold "constituent validity." Thus, the implications for training are two-fold. First, an array of research methods courses, both qualitative and quantitative should be part of training, particularly at the doctoral level. Second, the courses should focus not only on the acquisition of technical skills in design, data collection, and analysis but also on developing creative problem solving skills in contouring designs to fit with community input and social ecology principles (that is, multiple interventions at multiple social levels).

Possible Institutional Consequences for University-Based Researchers

CBPR takes time. Researchers and practitioners must be responsive both to the slow and deliberate pace that often accompanies community engagement and to the pressures and timelines programs and schools of public health maintain for promotion and tenure. If expectations regarding scholarly productivity are not met, those early in their careers may soon be out of a job. The irony is that those who become well-mentored in CBPR may not have the opportunity to build upon years of productive partnering because they do not pass muster at the university. If CBPR and practice are to be established as core methods in public health, then reward and incentive systems for faculty promotion and tenure may require adjustments to accommodate the complex nature of the work.

Community-based research involves active partnerships between the community and researchers. These partnerships are important to developing prevention research and health promotion programs because no single agency or institution has the resources, access, and trust relationships to address the wide range of community determinants of public health problems (Green and Mercer, 2001). Public health professionals in the 21st century must understand the major concepts and principles underlying community-based research to engage more effectively in research and practice activities.

GLOBAL HEALTH

America has a vital and direct stake in the health of people around the globe, and . . . this interest derives from both America's long and enduring tradition of humanitarian concern and compelling reasons of enlightened self-interest (IOM, 1997).

It is clear that health concerns and interventions cannot be limited by national borders. Increased travel, migration, and refugees from conflict have had an impact on the demographics of the United States. It is not unusual for a local U.S. community to be composed of immigrants from many areas of the globe with different cultural traditions and beliefs. The extent to which these immigrants adjust well to life in the United States and experience healthy development depends on several things, including (1) the assets and resources they bring from their country of origin, (2) how they are officially categorized and treated by federal, state, and local governments, (3) the social and economic circumstances and cultural environment in which they reside in the U.S., and (4) the treatment they receive from other individuals and from health and social institutions in the receiving community (IOM, 1998). These rapidly growing immigrant communities are creating a need for new services or for providing old services in a way that takes into account the traditions and beliefs of the different cultures.

There is a growing need to address issues that impact global health, such as the increasing income differentials between and among countries that foster poverty-associated conditions for poor health; the variance in environmental and occupational health and safety standards that contributes to hazardous production facilities and dangerous working conditions; global environmental changes leading to such things as depletion of freshwater supplies and the loss of arable lands; and the re-emergence of infectious diseases (IOM, 1997; McMichael and Beaglehole, 2000).

Poverty and ill health have long been associated, and the number of poor and marginalized people is increasing (Macfarlane et al., 2000). For every 100,000 births in developing regions, 500 women die as a result of pregnancy and childbirth while the rich countries have a rate of 7 maternal deaths per 100,000 births (IOM, 1997). Poverty contributes to population growth, which, in turn, leads to overcrowded and unsanitary living conditions in poor communities which, in turn, leads to the spread of infectious diseases. HIV/AIDS and tuberculosis continue to cause substantial numbers of deaths in many developing countries. Other diseases such as malaria, dengue, and cholera are re-emerging. Table 3-2, outlines factors contributing to disease reemergence.

Overpopulation also affects the environment. "Humankind is now disrupting at a global level some of the biosphere's life-support systems," for example, changing the composition of the atmosphere and depleting ocean fisheries (McMichael and Beaglehole, 2000). With increasing population comes a need for increased food production. However erosion, compaction, salination, waterlogging, and chemicalization that destroys organic content have damaged an estimated one-third of the world's previously productive land (McMichael and Beaglehole, 2000).

Some multinational companies, taking advantage of cross-national variations in environmental and worker safety standards, place hazardous production facilities in developing countries that either do not have strict regulations governing such facilities or that have lax enforcement. Lee (1999) quotes Deacon as saying "[E]conomic competition between countries may be leading them to shed the economic costs of social protection in order to be more competitive (social dumping) unless there are supranational or global regulations in place that discourage this." The result of this social dumping has, according to Lee, been a long-term deterioration of public health systems, including the ability to manage infectious diseases. Additionally, pollution has caused the creation of "hot zones" that are believed to have led to a new strain of *Vibrio Cholerae* that may be starting the world's eighth cholera pandemic (Epstein, 1992).

Issues related to food safety and diet are also of global concern. According to Kickbusch and Buse (2001), "A 300 percent increase in the real

TABLE 3-2   Factors Contributing to Disease Reemergence and Examples of Associated Infections

Contributing Factors	Associated Infectious Diseases
Human demographics and behavior	Dengue/dengue hemorrhagic fever, sexually transmitted diseases, giardiasis
Technology and industry	Toxic shock syndrome, nosocomial (hospital acquired) infections, hemorrhagic colitis/ hemolytic uremic syndrome
Economic development and land use	Lyme disease, malaria, plague, rabies, yellow fever, Rift Valley fever, schistosomiasis
International travel and commerce	Malaria, cholera, pneumococcal pneumonia
Microbial adaptation and change	Influenza, HIV/AIDS, malaria, Staphlococcus aureus infections
Breakdown of public health measures	Rabies, tuberculosis, trench fever, diphtheria, whooping cough (pertussis), cholera

SOURCE: IOM, 1997.

value of the global trade in food between 1974 and 1994 (Kaferstein et al., 1997), coupled with increased travel and changes in lifestyles and nutrition patterns, demographics and vulnerability, and microbial populations, all intertwine to create a new pattern of susceptibility." The recent European concern over "mad cow disease" in English beef is an illustration in point.

The transfer of unhealthy diets (e.g., high fat) and unsafe products (e.g., tobacco and firearms) are also relevant to global health. For example, the decline in smoking in western countries has been accompanied by massive marketing and increased smoking rates in low- and middle-income countries. It is estimated that one-third of Chinese males under age 30 will be killed by tobacco and about 22 percent of all deaths in Eastern Europe will be related to smoking by the year 2020 (Kickbusch and Buse, 2001).

Another area of concern is preparedness against bioterrorism. Since the anthrax attacks of September 2001, there has been heightened awareness of the possiblity of bioterrorism. International surveillance and safeguards against man-made infectious outbreaks are in the process of being strengthened. Public health professionals of the 21st century must be better prepared to respond in the face of such attacks, including understanding the actions available to them to respond and the authorities under which those actions can be taken.

Global health challenges are increasingly important. Many of these challenges are beyond the scope of this report. However, the committee believes that public health professionals must understand global health issues and their determinants; they must understand how local actions can have health impacts across the globe. Public health must be prepared to work with individuals from other countries to solve the problems facing our global community. To effectively engage with others on an international basis will require not only knowledge and skills described under the other seven content areas discussed in this chapter, but also an ecological perspective of the determinants of health.

We are all on this planet together. It behooves us to care for the natural and human resources so vital to the existence of us all.

POLICY AND LAW

Although the importance of policy in public health has long been recognized (IOM, 1988), education in policy and law at many programs and schools of public health is currently minimal. Education in policy analysis and, in particular, in policy methods, needs to be strengthened and systematically provided to all students, consistent with the inclusion of policy development as a core competency for public health professionals (Council on Linkages, 2001).

Turnock (2001) writes that "policy development involves serving the public interest in the development of comprehensive public health outcomes by promoting the use of the scientific knowledge base in decision making and by leading in developing public health policy." The pace of policy development is poorly matched with the pace of scientific research, however. Policy-makers are accustomed to making decisions based on incomplete information; public health professionals can be a more effective part of that process if they are familiar and equipped with reliable data produced on a shorter time frame. It is also important to recognize the underlying difficulty that choices based upon incomplete information are inevitable and that our programs and schools of public health are not doing a particularly good job of educating students to manage the associated uncertainties. Educating students in traditional epidemiologic and biostatistical methods is important, but in addition to those methods, students also need training in quantitative methods (e.g., decision analysis, policy modeling, Bayesian statistics) aimed at promoting better policy decisions under conditions of uncertainty.

Engagement in policy also requires a set of practical political skills (IOM, 1988; Gebbie and Hwang, 2000). Successful community public health work at the policy level typically requires political collaboration with stakeholders (Freudenberg and Golub, 1987). Public health professionals in the community can be more effective if they can understand the dynamics of community politics, identify and work with stakeholders, identify legal and policy structures currently influencing community health and efficacy, and motivate and educate stakeholders and officials.

These skills can be taught to some extent, but also require "interdisciplinary dialogue, faculty modeling of political competence; opportunities for students to realize personal, professional, and political connections; and a concern of socialization in the context of global citizenship" (Rains and Barton-Kriese, 2001). People in practice report the need for more skills in policy development and law (Liang et al., 1993).

Law is an essential component of training in policy. Most public health policies are embodied in or effectuated through law, and law provides the institutional framework and procedures through which policies are debated, codified, implemented, and interpreted (Burris, 1994; Gostin, 2000). Law is more than just the rules written down in statutes and court decisions; it encompasses the institutional arrangements and day-to-day practices through which law influences behavior and attitudes (Ewick and Silbey, 1998; Sarat, 1990; Burris, 2002). The effectiveness of public health leaders at the local, state or national level will be significantly enhanced by knowledge about law including its structure, its typical modes of operation, the powers (and the limitations on power) provided for public health actions, and its role in population health and behavior. These domains have been embodied in a set of core legal competencies, prepared by the Center for Law and the Public's Health with support from CDC.

A critical area in public health policy research is engagement with law. Within the ecological model of health, laws and legal practices may be important constituents of the "fundamental social causes of disease" that broadly determine population vulnerability and immunity from illness (Link and Phelan, 1995; Sweat, 1995; Burris et al., 2002; Sumartojo, 2000). Public health research seeking to understand the relationship of multiple determinants of health will be enhanced by integrating law and legal practices into research on individuals, partners, communities, and whole populations. Because laws are used as structural interventions to regulate individual behavior and to change social and material conditions that endanger health (Blankenship, 2000; Hemenway, 2001; Schmid et al., 1995), law is also an important tool for intervention in public health, and here research has a vital role to play.

Research in public health can help to document how health policy is made (and the process influenced) (Backstrom and Robins, 1995; Mittelmark, 1999), as well as the difference between law on the books and law in practice (Boden, 1996; Cotton-Oldenburg, 2001). The challenge is not only to recognize law as a part of the universe of factors to be studied, but also to develop and support methods that are appropriate to the study of law's operation in a population over time. The operation of law cannot often be studied in experimental designs. More attention to and respect for observational studies, rapid assessments, qualitative methods, and modeling is essential to expanding the public health research base in law.

Major barriers to increasing law-related research in public health are lack of funding and faculty incentives for efforts to make research more useful in the policy process (Nutbeam, 1996). Historically, funding for law-related research in public health has been minimal. In recent years, the CDC has made an important commitment to funding public health law research, but awareness of and support for this field of work remains rare in the National Institutes of Health.

Ethics, too, play an important role in politics and policy development as elsewhere in practice. Ethics are a tool through which public health professionals can interrogate their own values, formulate policy goals, and articulate a rationale for change in policy. Gostin suggests that

> [p]ublic health ethics . . . can illuminate the field of public health in several ways. Ethics can offer guidance on (i) the meaning of public health professionalism and the ethical practice of the profession; (ii) the moral weight and value of the community's health and wellbeing; (iii) the recurring themes of the field and the dilemmas faced in everyday public health practice; and (iv) the role of advocacy to achieve the goal of safer and healthier populations (Gostin, 2002).

While the content of public health ethics will continue to develop, the committee believes that ethics are an important and heretofore neglected element of a thorough education in policy.

Finally, policy training in programs and schools of public health also can be enhanced by considering human rights and their relation to health. As used in public health circles, human rights cut across law, ethics, and advocacy. When evoked in terms of the various international human rights conventions and national constitutions, they are a species of law (Burris, 2002). As deployed in efforts to secure just and effective public health policies, they are a tool of advocacy (Gostin and Lazzarini, 1997). Jonathan Mann argued that human rights could also take the place of an ethics for public health (Mann, 1997). While much work remains to be done to develop the public health potential of human rights analysis (Gostin, 2002), a human rights perspective has already become an important part of international health practice.

ETHICS[1]

Public health raises a number of moral problems that extend beyond the earlier boundaries of bioethics and require their own form of ethical analysis (Callahan and Jennings, 2002).

Ethics, in general terms, are "values or standards designed to shed light on the relative rightness or wrongness of actions based on moral principles, professionally endorsed and practiced" (Modeste, 1996). Public health is confronted with a wide array of ethical issues and questions, including issues involving: advances in technology and how they will be applied to improve the health of populations (e.g., information technology and genomics), the decisions we make about what and how to communicate, the ways in which we interact with diverse populations, the extent to which we develop partnerships and collaboration for public health programs and research, and resource allocation for provision of care.

The ethical basis for the practice of the health professions has been well studied by both health professionals and ethicists for some time. A statement of public health practice ethics has only recently been produced, and very little attention is paid to public health ethics in educational programs. Few schools of public health have trained ethicists on faculty, despite the fact that 22 of the 25 responding schools of public health report teaching ethics. To foster appropriate thinking and action

---

[1]Much of the material in this section is abstracted from the commissioned paper prepared for the committee by James C. Thomas, M.P.H., Ph.D.

in public health, with its immense potential to influence populations, research and teaching in ethics as they apply to public health must be strengthened.

Callahan and Jennings (2002) have described the scope of issues in public health ethics as encompassing four general categories: health promotion and disease prevention, risk reduction, epidemiological and other public health research, and structural and socioeconomic disparities. They further identify different types of ethical analysis: professional ethics, applied ethics, advocacy ethics, and critical ethics, and they encourage all schools of public health to promote the teaching of ethics.

The American Public Health Association (APHA) has recently adopted a public health code of ethics (see Box 3-1). This code is based upon certain identified values and beliefs of public health including:

- a belief in the interdependence of people and between people and their environment,
  - the importance of addressing root causes of health and illness,
  - the utility of the scientific method for gaining information, and
  - the importance of acting on reliable information that is in hand when the resources are available to do so (Thomas et al., 2002).

Public health ethics differs from medical ethics, which is typically concerned with an individual who is ill or disabled. Part of the ethical equation in medicine is whether withholding a treatment is tantamount to failing to rescue a person when rescue is possible. Moreover, the risks of introducing an intervention may be more palatable in view of the suffering that is likely in the absence of the intervention. In the case of public health prevention,[2] however, the person or population is not necessarily ill or disabled, and the potential benefits of an intervention are less salient to those who might experience them. Even after an intervention to prevent an illness or injury is in place, benefits are often invisible or at least not in the forefront of people's minds. Seldom do people think, for example, of the illnesses they did not get because they were vaccinated, or the cavities they did not have because the water supply was fluoridated. The hidden nature of some prevention benefits places an extra burden on public health professionals to clarify to the public the benefits of an intervention and how those benefits outweigh the risks of not intervening.

---

[2] Prevention can be categorized into three types: primary, secondary, and tertiary. Primary prevention, to which this statement refers, is the prevention of an illness or a disability. Secondary prevention is the treatment of a curable illness, and is designed to limit the progression of an illness or a disability. In the case of irreversible conditions, tertiary prevention is prevention of the progression to a more serious illness or disability, or the postponement of death.

BOX 3-1   Principles of the Ethical Practice of Public Health

1. Public health should address principally the fundamental causes of disease and requirements for health, aiming to prevent adverse health outcomes.
2. Public health should achieve community health in a way that respects the rights of individuals in the community.
3. Public health policies, programs, and priorities should be developed and evaluated through processes that ensure an opportunity for input from community members.
4. Public health should advocate for, or work for the empowerment of, disenfranchised community members, ensuring that the basic resources and conditions necessary for health are accessible to all people in the community.
5. Public health should seek the information needed to implement effective policies and programs that protect and promote health.
6. Public health institutions should provide communities with the information they have that is needed for decisions on policies or programs and should obtain the community's consent for their implementation.
7. Public health institutions should act in a timely manner on the information they have within the resources and the mandate given to them by the public.
8. Public health programs and policies should incorporate a variety of approaches that anticipate and respect diverse values, beliefs, and cultures in the community.
9. Public health programs and policies should be implemented in a manner that most enhances the physical and social environment.
10. Public health institutions should protect the confidentiality of information that can bring harm to an individual or community if made public. Exceptions must be justified on the basis of the high likelihood of significant harm to the individual or others.
11. Public health institutions should ensure the professional competence of their employees.
12. Public health institutions and their employees should engage in collaborations and affiliations in ways that build the public's trust and the institution's effectiveness.

SOURCE: Thomas et al., 2002. Reprinted with permission of *Am J Public Health*, 2002; 7: 1057–9.

The public health focus on populations also differs from the medical focus on interactions between a patient and a care provider. With a population perspective, public health institutions think in terms of healthy populations and communities as well as healthy individuals. The health of a community includes the quality of interactions among community members (consider, for example, the prevention of violence) and among institutions serving the community (e.g., the need for collaboration to achieve complex goals). A community perspective thus highlights the interdependence of individuals and organizations. This stands in contrast to the importance given to autonomy in medical ethics, in which the concern is principally to prevent a patient from being abused by a care provider who wields much power. Although personal autonomy remains an important consideration in public health ethics, it is counterbalanced by concern for the well-being of a whole population and a realization that not everyone affected by a particular public health action will agree with it. Thus, in public health the personal choices and preferences of some will be overridden by a greater concern for the well-being of a whole population.

Policies and practices affecting a population are typically designed and implemented by government and other organizations, raising the question of how an agency develops and maintains an ethical compass. Is it through policy-making, or, in the case of governmental agencies, through legislation? Does it include understandings within a community that transcend legislation (e.g., a concern for equal access that is not legally mandated)? How are ethical conundrums resolved or decisions made in an organization that includes employees with different perspectives and sensibilities? An important part of public health ethics is sorting through ethical issues in a group setting.

The combination of a population perspective and institutional action presents a particular ethical danger to public health. "Population" and "institution" are abstract concepts, neither of which bears a human face. The ability to sympathize with another is a fundamental aspect of being able to think and act ethically towards that person. Personal interactions can lead to sympathy. However, interactions between an institution and a population occur in such a way that sympathy is not a common element of the interaction. To an epidemiologist, the population may be represented as a data set. Even to a public health ethicist, thinking about a population may be an exercise in wrestling with other abstract concepts such as the distribution of scarce resources. All too frequently such an exercise does not stem from direct interaction with those who will be most affected by a decision regarding those resources.

From the perspective of the individual in the community, the public health institution also lacks a human face. In this situation, however, the primary concern resulting from the impersonal nature of the institution is not the ethical treatment of the institution by individuals but the ability of individuals to trust the institution. A widespread absence of trust can severely limit the effectiveness of the institution. Ethical treatment of an individual and community by the institution, however, builds trust. In this way, the ethical functioning of a public health institution also affects its effectiveness in accomplishing its mission.

Public health needs both scholars who can articulate the unique aspects of public health ethics and public health practitioners who understand and operate within the ethics structures of the field. Nancy Kass (2001) discusses a six-step ethics framework for public health that can serve as an analytic tool used to help consider ethical implications of proposed interventions, policies, research, and programs. The six steps are as follows:

1) What are the public health goals of the proposed program?
2) How effective is the program in achieving its stated goals?
3) What are the known or potential burdens of the program?
4) Can burdens be minimized? Are there alternative approaches?
5) Is the program implemented fairly?
6) How can the benefits and burdens of a program be fairly balanced?

Thomas, in the paper prepared for this committee, identified seven areas for education in public health ethics. First, are *the values and beliefs inherent to a public health perspective.* A list of these was developed in conjunction with the Public Health Code of Ethics (Thomas et al., 2002). They are presented on the Web at www.apha.org/codeofethics and include: a belief in the interdependence of people and between people and their environment; the importance of addressing root causes of health and illness; the use of the scientific method for gaining information; and the importance of acting upon reliable information when the resources are available to do so.

Secondly, education in public health ethics should address *ethical principles that follow from the values and beliefs outlined above.* The Public Health Code of Ethics consists of 12 ethical principles (see Box 3-1) that address the relationship between public health institutions and the populations they serve. Other codes of ethics for epidemiology and health education provide additional information more specific to these practices (located on the Web, respectively, at www.acepidemiology.org/policystmts/EthicsGuide.htm and www.sophe.org/).

Public health mandates and powers is another important component of education. Students should understand the legal mandates given to public health institutions and the powers available to them to meet the mandates and the potential abuses of these powers. It is also important to know that the powers of non-public-health organizations, such as some private companies, affect the health of the public and to consider how public health ethics might extend to them.

Further, *ethical tensions within public health* should be included in an understanding of public health ethics. Some ethical questions arise frequently because of an underlying, irresolvable tension between ethical principles. One that is common in public health is the tension between the need to protect the health of an entire community and the need to honor the rights of individuals in the community. This tension is brought to the fore when an individual claims that a public health regulation violates his or her rights. Examples of how some of these situations have been handled can be helpful in navigating future conflicts.

It is important to review *historical ethical failures and triumphs*. One ethical failure in public health was the study of syphilis that was conducted by the Public Health Service and the Tuskegee Institute. Students should be aware of this study and what went wrong. It is also important to provide examples of ethical triumphs and more modest failures. An exclusive focus on "monstrous" failures can lead some to believe that ethics are not a concern for "normal" people such as themselves.

Two other areas to include are *the history and purposes of research ethics institutions* and *the application of ethics to specific topics such as informatics and genomics*. Institutional Review Boards (IRBs) currently review research proposals to ensure that they are consistent with rules and regulations concerning human experimentation. It is imperative that public health researchers and practitioners know how to interact with such boards and appreciate the value of this review system. In terms of specific topics, much of contemporary practical ethics is driven by new technological developments. The use of information about individuals that can be managed through sophisticated electronic systems, and in some instances acquired through genetic tools are two that bear directly on public health and affect nearly every public health practitioner. Students need to be informed of the prevalent ethical standards for using these tools.

"Ethical analysis can further understanding in every area of public health practice" (Levin, 2002), and it is essential that programs and schools of public health incorporate the teaching of ethics. However, the barriers to teaching ethics are substantial and, if not required, it is likely that ethics will not be taught in any meaningful way. Requiring ethics instruction in the curriculum does not necessarily mean requiring a free-standing course. A free-standing course entitled "ethics" might unintentionally convey the notion that ethics stands apart from other topics in public health, as opposed to the notion that it permeates every topic. Conversely, sometimes ethics teaching is best received when it is not billed as ethics. For example, a course may include instruction in how to interact with community members and thus communicate the importance of community input without appealing to it explicitly as an ethical principle.

There are dangers in not creating a free-standing course in ethics, however. In the absence of a required course, individual courses are likely to include an ethics lecture or two. Unless there is some coordination among courses, they are likely to cover similar material. A student may thus sit through three lectures on the Tuskegee study of syphilis or the functions of an IRB, but never learn to reason through tensions between individual interests and the good of the community or how to avoid unethical conflicts of interest. An uncoordinated ethics curriculum can easily be neither broad nor deep; it can be an inch wide and an inch deep.

However a program or school chooses to integrate ethics, a necessary first step is to identify competencies in public health ethics. Once the core competencies are identified, a curriculum committee can ensure that they are covered within the required courses, regardless of whether a topic is labeled as ethics when it is taught.

The committee recognizes that teaching ethics in programs and schools of public health requires faculty educated to do so. This means that faculty will, themselves, require education in ethics, and schools and programs will need to provide professional incentives and rewards that encourage and value ethics as a subject of teaching and research.

Ethics is most stale and irrelevant when it is solely academic. Ethics is something less than ethics when it is not put into practice. Putting ethics into practice means that ethics should not be limited to a list of rules and regulations. Although these often represent the encoding of the ethical values of an institution, they are seldom adequate to address all situations, and they will never obviate the need for individuals and groups to have skills in reasoning through ethical conundrums.

It is also important that classroom teaching on ethics be linked to practical, real-life situations. Ideally, this might involve site visits to various neighborhoods or discussions with study participants. To counter the dehumanizing potential of a population perspective, mentioned above, public health students need to interact with individuals who are most affected by a particular ethical decision.

Regardless of whether ethics is taught explicitly, ethical values are communicated though teaching, mentoring, public health research and interventions, interactions between the school and other institutions, and more. If not taught explicitly, the accidental teaching of ethics is likely to be inconsistent and nonsystematic, and may perpetuate unethical actions. To promote ethical practices and to prepare students for the multitude of ethical decisions they will confront, students must be taught ethics in an intentional way. The means by which this is done, whether in a free-standing course or integrated into the curriculum, is less important than the identification of competencies along with a system of ensuring that these competencies are fully covered in the curriculum. To facilitate the teaching of ethics, schools and programs must institutionalize incentives for faculty to develop interest in ethics and the ability to teach the topic. For the teaching of ethics to be credible and vital to students, ethical education must include a practical component, most likely in the field, and schools and programs of public health education must personify a high ethical standard.

Law is another emerging area for public health scholarship, and while ethics and law are often discussed as related fields, each deserves attention in its own right. However, law overlaps with ethics, in that public health laws themselves should be ethical, as should the implementation of those laws. Since law can influence the social and physical environment in ways that are important to health, it is much more than a set of rules; law also encompasses the institutions and practices that bring these rules to daily life. Understanding this ethical perspective of law and using law in this way requires much more than mastery of regulations about specific businesses (restaurants, water systems) and the administrative procedures through which they are administered, though these are important. It brings to the forefront the use of law to influence choices made by individuals through the rewards or penalties that accrue.

SUMMARY

Each of the eight content areas discussed in this chapter is important for the future of public health and public health education. Understanding and being able to apply information and computer science technology to public health practice and learning (i.e., public health informatics) are crucial competencies for public health professionals in this information age in which we are vitally dependent upon data and information. Genomics is helping us understand the causative role of genetic factors in leading causes of morbidity in the United States, information that is important to the ecological model public health professionals must use to better understand how to improve health. Public health professionals must be proficient in communication in order to interact effectively with multiple audiences. They also must be able to understand and incorporate the needs and perspectives of culturally diverse communities in public health interventions and research. New approaches to research that involve practitioners, researchers, and the community in joint efforts to improve health are becoming more necessary as we recognize the importance of the impact of multiple determinants on health, for example, social relationships, living conditions, neighborhoods, and communities. Understanding global health issues is increasingly important as public health professionals are called upon to address problems that transcend national boundaries. Public health professionals must also understand how best to inform policy makers as they develop policies, laws, and regulations that have an impact on the public's health. Finally, public health professionals must be able to identify and address the numerous ethical issues that arise in public health practice and research.

Therefore, **for each of these eight emerging content areas, the committee recommends that:**

- **competencies be identified;**
- **each area be included in graduate level public health education;**
- **continuing development and creation of new knowledge be pursued; and**
- **opportunity for specialization be offered.**

The committee has highlighted the importance of these eight areas because it believes that they are and will continue to be central to public health for some time to come. It is beyond the charge of this committee to prepare curricula for educating public health professionals in these areas, yet it is crucial that such curricula be developed. As our understanding evolves, and as conditions change, other new knowledge and skills will be identified that will need to be incorporated into public health professional education. The committee emphasizes that it is important that public health education not "freeze" with the focus as identified in this report. Rather, the committee believes that the progress made in understanding and incorporating these eight important areas into public health practice, education, and research will enable us, in the future, to identify other new and emerging areas that must be addressed.

The committee also believes that it is important to enhance the development of the profession of public health, with some advocating the use of credentialing and certification as approaches to workforce development. Credentialing is a formal process used to ensure that persons practicing in a profession meet minimum standards (Modeste, 1996). Certification is "a process by which a quasi-governmental agency or association grants recognition or licensure to a person who has met certain qualifications specified by that agency. For example, the National Commission for Health Education Credentialing (NCHEC) certifies health educators. CDC and other public health agencies and organizations such as the National Association of County and City Health Officers (NACCHO), ASPH, and APHA are examining the feasibility of creating a credentialing system for public health. Their efforts are focused on credentialing based on competencies linked to the essential public health services framework.

Many issues that need to be pursued in this area are beyond the scope of this report. Certification, however, relates to the education of public health professionals. Within the various professions in the world of health and illness, the process of certification is common. In some cases, such as medicine and nursing, specialty certification is available only to those who have first qualified for a license to practice that is granted by a state authority. The specialty certification attests to skills beyond the legal minimum that apply to a limited set of patients (e.g., pediatrics), conditions (e.g., infectious diseases), or interventions (e.g., anesthesia). There are also areas of practice for which there is no required state licensure but for which members of the practice field have created certification as a way of attesting to minimum or common capacities. In public health, perhaps the best known is the Certified Health Education Specialist (CHES). In environmental health, there is also the mixed model of the registered sanitarian, who may be certified by the National Environmental Health Association but is required to achieve a state license in some states.

The range of individuals entering M.P.H. programs, many with no previous health-specific education and with no access to the public health-related certifications currently in existence, makes this group likely candidates for a certification program. Defining specific criteria for such certification as well as designating a responsible organization to carry out out the process is beyond the scope of this report. However, the committee believes that voluntary certification for the M.P.H. graduate would enhance the profession. Therefore, **the committee recommends the development of a *voluntary* certification of competence in the ecological approach to public health as a mechanism for encouraging the development of new M.P.H. graduates.**

This chapter has described the future of public health professional education, no matter the site at which that education is obtained. Chapter 4 discusses the role of schools of public health in educating public health professionals, while Chapter 5 discusses the roles of other schools and programs. Chapter 6 focuses on the state, local, and federal public health agencies.

4

Future Role of Schools of Public Health in Educating Public Health Professionals for the 21st Century

OVERVIEW

The history of education in schools of public health has been one of evolution and change in response to new knowledge, the needs of the times, and opportunities for improvement. Schools are again faced with the need to evolve, in part because current problems demand new knowledge and approaches, and in part because of scientific advances and the increased understanding of the determinants of health, their linkages, and their interactions. Faculty in schools of public health come from multiple disciplines, making schools uniquely poised to embrace the transdisciplinary approach to education and research that is necessary for an ecological focus. The ecological model for public health discussed in Chapter 1 provides a focus for the following discussion, a discussion that identifies responsibilities, explores future directions, and makes recommendations for strengthening education, research, and training in schools of public health.

The committee determined that schools of public health have six major responsibilities. These are to:

1) educate the educators, practitioners, and researchers as well as to prepare public health leaders and managers;

2) serve as a focal point for multi-school transdisciplinary research as well as traditional public health research to improve the health of the public;

3) contribute to policy that advances the health of the public;

4) work collaboratively with other professional schools to assure quality public health content in their programs;

5) assure access to life-long learning for the public health workforce; and

6) engage actively with various communities to improve the public's health.

The following pages discuss each of these responsibilities and provide recommendations for a framework for education, training, and research in schools of public health.

EDUCATION

The "most distinctive role of public health education lies in the preparation of public health professionals" (Fineberg et al., 1994). While most professional public health graduates receive their degrees in either 1 of the 32 accredited schools of public health (about 5,600 graduates in 1999) or 1 of the 45 accredited master of public health (M.P.H.) degree programs (approximately 800 graduates in 2001), it has been amply documented that only a small minority of the total public health workforce has received *any* formal public health training. In an 18-month study of the Texas public health workforce, Kennedy and colleagues (1999) estimated that only 7 percent of the public health workforce had formal education in public health. Nationally, only 22 percent of chief executives of local health departments have graduate degrees in public health (Turnock, 2001), and it is estimated that about 80 percent of public health workers lack basic training in public health (CDC, 2001a).

Many of those in the public health *workforce* who do receive formal training in public health do so primarily via alternative pathways, that is, through certificate programs, short courses, and continuing education programs, conferences, workshops, and institutes offered by a variety of institutions and organizations. The strengths and contributions of these programs cannot be overemphasized, and the committee acknowledges their importance to the development of the public health workforce.

The committee believes that education in schools of public health should be directed toward masters and doctoral level students who will fulfill many professional positions within public health, toward persons destined for practice careers in positions of senior responsibility and leadership, and toward those who will become public health researchers and academic faculty. The education and range of skills of professionals working in public health will continue to be wide. There is a need for well-educated senior public health officials who "have the preparation not only to manage a governmental agency, but also to provide guidance to the workforce with regard to health goals or priorities, provide policy direction to a governing board, and interact with other agencies, at all levels of government, whose actions and decisions affect the population whose health he or she is trying to assure" (Turnock, 2001). Schools of public health are in the ideal position to focus on this needed leadership development because of the range of skills and knowledge represented within the faculty, and because of the partnerships that can be sustained with public health practice. This focus can most effectively be done if it becomes a priority for educational programs.

This does not mean that schools of public health should see themselves as the only and exclusive training ground for leadership. Rather this education for senior-level responsibility in practice is important, and schools of public health should respond to the need for such education. Schools of public health will also continue to educate masters and doctoral level students to fill many professional positions within public health. Some schools will directly educate the broader public health workforce through curriculum setting, distance learning, cross training, and continuing education and other methods. However, **the committee recommends that schools embrace as a primary educational mission the preparation of individuals for positions of senior responsibility in public health practice, research, and teaching**. It is important for schools to emphasize responsibility to prepare future public health leaders. Both the selection of students and the approach to imparting knowledge, skills, and attitudes should be guided by this expectation. The challenges discussed in Chapter 1, and the eight important content areas described in Chapter 3, as well as other factors, speak to the need for attracting to schools of public health a wide range of students from numerous and varied populations and disciplines. Such diversity has the potential to strengthen the knowledge exchange among disciplines, moving us more rapidly toward a transdisciplinary approach to learning and an ecological model for action.

Currently, schools of public health base their curriculum on five core disciplines: epidemiology, biostatistics, environmental health sciences, health services administration, and social and behavioral sciences. Recently, the Council on Linkages Between Academia and Public Health Practice outlined a list of eight competency domains intended to strengthen education in some of these areas. The competency areas are:

1) analytic/assessment
2) policy development/program planning
3) communication
4) cultural competence
5) community dimensions of practice
6) basic public health sciences (namely, biostatistics, epidemiology, environmental health, health services administration, and social and behavioral sciences)

7) financial planning and management
8) leadership and systems thinking

The committee reaffirms the importance of the long recognized core areas (epidemiology, biostatistics, environmental health, health services administration, and social and behavioral sciences). Further, the committee endorses the idea that education should be competency based and supports educational programs built upon the competency domains identified by the Council on Linkages. However, public health professionals in the 21st century must also understand the ecological nature of the determinants of health, that is, their linkages and relationships. Such an understanding is necessary to design, implement, and evaluate public health interventions. Several critical gaps have been identified in the current approach to educating public health professionals. These gaps include informatics, genomics, community-based research, global health, law, and ethics. Additionally, the committee believes that greater emphasis must be placed upon the Council on Linkages' identified competency areas of communication, policy, and cultural competence. Finally, the committee believes that schools must carefully examine how their courses are structured and how learning is provided.

Therefore, **schools of public health should emphasize the importance and centrality of the ecological approach. Further, schools have a primary role in influencing the incorporation of this ecological view of public health, as well as a population focus, into all health professional education and practice.** The ecological approach and emphasis on public health practice require a careful examination of how courses and other elements of the program are structured. There are probably many new and innovative ways that will better facilitate particular areas of learning (e.g., policy development) than classroom-based lectures, for example, case-based learning (see example provided in Box 4-1). The committee encourages schools to examine alternatives to traditional teaching modes.

A comparison of the expanded areas of competency with current M.P.H. curricula at most U.S. institutions suggests substantial non-alignment. The present structure is heavily oriented toward teaching the basic public health sciences, augmented by specialization in one such area. Most of the education is didactic in nature; practical training is generally limited to community rotations of varying intensity. In addition, many curricula require an intensive research experience for completion of degree requirements, which is positive for those who envision careers in research, but less well-justified for those who engage in senior level practice positions. Teaching is conducted primarily by faculty with backgrounds in one of the core public health sciences. There is presently minimal participation in the educational process by those in senior practice positions or with comparable experiences, experts in medicine or its prac-

---

BOX 4-1 Case-Based Learning Example
West Nile Virus

You are health commissioner for a suburban county in a major metropolitan area. The previous summer several cases of encephalitis were diagnosed at area hospitals and identified as being caused by a hemorrhagic virus previously unknown in the region. Mortality, thankfully, was limited to a small number of very debilitated elderly patients. A combined effort of veterinarians, infectious disease specialists, and your colleagues documented that the virus had infected local crows (the reservoir) and was present in a high proportion of mosquitoes in the community. Efforts to control the mosquito population in neighboring towns, requiring extensive public spraying with pesticides, resulted in widespread complaints because of acute reactions to the chemicals among some chemically sensitive residents. Additionally, many environmentalists raised concerns about long term health effects of the chemicals used.

It is now April, and early tests reveal a high rate of infection in crows, as well as evidence that the mosquito population is again infested. The situation is further complicated by advice from the agricultural extension service in your community that the mosquito population is anticipated to be unusually large this season because of the warm, wet winter. Local community groups are duly worried: the environmentalists, about the possibility of toxic spraying; parent groups about the infectious risks to children from playing soccer, going to the beach, etc. Physicians in the community are concerned about encephalitis risk as well, especially among the elderly. As commissioner you must devise and defend a course of action.

TASKS
- What factual pieces of information do you need to devise an appropriate plan? How might you obtain them? What will you do if some/all are unavailable?
- What specific control strategies should be considered, separately or together?
- What infrastructure(s) would need to be in place to implement these strategies? What would you do about those which are not?
- How will you manage the competing concerns of the interested parties?
- Once you have selected an approach, what factors need to be considered for implementation?
- How do you plan to assess the effectiveness of your choice(s)?
- Under what circumstances would you modify your initial plan?

---

tice, or those with unique skills in areas such as communication, cultural competence, leadership development, or planning. The following sections highlight strategies and recommendations to achieve the proposed realignment. In addition, the allocation of appropriate financial resources to achieve these proposals is essential. Recommendations for funding appear in Chapter 6.

Educating Leaders in Public Health Practice

Successful transition to programs with appropriate emphasis, faculty, and teaching approaches consistent with the proposed competencies will require radical change. First and foremost, since the goal is to inculcate a broad ecologic perspective, and the sheer amount of content material is increasingly vast, integrative teaching techniques (such as case-based learning) may prove more appropriate than the traditional single discipline courses. Consideration may need to be given to upgrading the M.P.H. admissions requirements to ensure a high level of knowledge in basic science areas such as human biology, math, computer literacy, and environmental science. Second, the practical intention of the training would suggest that classroom teaching be substituted to the extent feasible by hands-on "rotations" with agencies and organizations of the type in which trainees are being prepared to function, including private sector organizations. Although long the preferred method for training physicians in preventive medicine, supervised, responsible, highly intensive and diverse experiences covering a gamut of public health settings are not currently available at most schools of public health. Implementation of increased "rotations" will require schools to develop and maintain relationships with the agencies and organizations that could serve as the practice sites.

Therefore, the committee recommends a significant expansion of *supervised* practice opportunities and sites (e.g., community-based public health programs, delivery systems, and health agencies). Such field work must be organized and supervised by faculty who have appropriate practical experience.

Problems with emphasizing the practice component in education delivered in schools of public health include lack of funding for quality practice experiences and the incentive and reward structures for academic faculty that do not reward practice scholarship. Academic institutions need to recognize faculty scholarship related to public health practice and service activities. Further, potential practice sites must be ready to receive and supervise public health students. This requires adequate funding for such activity, including training of practice site staff. Recommendations for such funding are discussed in Chapter 6, under the federal agency responsibility for public health education.

Many senior positions in public health will continue to demand or attract physicians, trained managers, lawyers, and others without formal public health training. Streamlined variations of the new practice curriculum that are oriented toward these individuals who have already obtained an M.D. (doctor of medicine), J.D. (doctor of law), M.B.A. (master of business administration) degree, or the equivalent will need to be developed to inculcate the core public health competencies in a practicable fashion as is currently done in preventive medicine training. Joint degrees in public health and these disciplines might be offered by universities with the appropriate schools and resources, as is currently the case on many campuses. Ideally such training might be incorporated into the medical school curriculum itself, as has been proposed by Lasker (1999) and others and is further discussed in Chapter 5 of this report.

The committee recommends that schools of public health should embrace the large number of programs in public-health-related fields that have developed within medical schools and schools of nursing, and initiate and foster scientific and educational collaborations.

The focus on preparing individuals for leadership roles and senior practice positions requires re-design of curricula and teaching approaches to incorporate:

- enhanced participation in the educational process by persons in senior practice positions or with comparable experiences, experts in medicine or its practice, or those with unique skills in areas such as communication, cultural competence, leadership development, policy, or planning;
- reconsideration of M.P.H. admission requirements to ensure that selected candidates are adequately prepared for the expanded didactic and practical training envisioned;
- vastly expanded practice rotations; and
- enhanced education for competence in specific careers (e.g., biostatistician or health care administrator).

Educating Public Health Researchers

As discussed later in this chapter, the range of future research in public health will also be radically different from what we see today. To a far greater degree, public health research will be transdisciplinary in nature, involving applications of basic biology and social sciences, and direct participation of the community. Moreover, a far larger portion of the research portfolio is likely to be evaluative and/or intervention-focused, with interventions at the individual, community organizational, and even societal levels.

Training of the workforce to conduct this research will require an equally radical new approach to the current strategy of advanced degree education at the doctoral level. The breadth of the envisioned future enterprise, and its many intersections with other scientific, biomedical, and social scientific fields, suggests that an important component of science training will be directed at those who enter public health with an advanced degree in another discipline, typically an M.D. or Ph.D. Such future investigators should have exposure to the core competencies and specialized advanced courses in relevant disciplines such as epidemiologic methods, methods for intervention research, or health economics. These types of courses may be necessary to transform the prior disciplinary research focus of these students to a new focus on public health questions. Efforts to make the educational experience efficient and flexible, as well as identifying sources to make this training economically feasible will be major determinants of success. For a variety of reasons, it may make sense for only some selected schools of public health—presumably those with a high base of external research activity and support—to perform this educational function, possibly even on a specialty-by-specialty basis. In other words, the several centers with advanced capability in international research methods might serve as "magnets" for this training; the handful with broad research expertise in occupational and environmental health sciences might do likewise for that field.

At the same time, some individuals may choose to obtain their primary doctoral level education at a school of public health. Doctoral candidates might be expected to have mastered undergraduate courses such as probability and statistics, computer applications, chemistry, biology, and human biology as prerequisites for admission directly into a doctoral program. In addition, given the intent for research training, such students would require external support throughout their education comparable to graduate students in other research-focused careers. Research training must not be construed as professional education geared toward practice in a high paying biomedical profession if the ambition is to train scientists.

The committee recommends that doctoral research training in public health should include an understanding of the multiple determinants of health within the ecological model. Doctoral research candidates should have exposure to core public health disciplines as well as areas identified as critical gaps in earlier discussion in this chapter, and researchers must be trained to understand communities and to engage in transdisciplinary research (see the section on transdisciplinary research).

Collaboration with Non-Traditional Programs

As discussed earlier, devising and implementing interventions that address the multiple determinants of health require interdisciplinary and multidisciplinary cooperation. Public health as a discipline and as a profession must be collaborative with other disciplines and professions, especially those within the broad health arena. Its modes of thinking and its distinct competencies must be applied across a range of organizations that exist within the community, especially those organizations that are directly concerned with, and have an impact on, health care and the health of the community's population.

The disciplines with which public health professionals must collaborate are, of course, not limited to health practitioners. They include lawyers, social workers, educators, housing specialists, community planners, and administrators of assisted-living facilities, to name a few. In a special way, those with whom public health must collaborate include health care practitioners such as physicians, nurses, physical therapists, occupational therapists, speech pathologists, audiologists, and dentists. Necessary collaboration will be enhanced to the extent that public health educators and students have the opportunity to meet with and share philosophical and methodological perspectives with educators and students in other professions.

Moreover, education toward collaboration will be enhanced and perhaps even maximized to the extent that other professionals can be educated within a school of public health. As students within a particular professional discipline, they will be required to follow a curriculum prescribed by national accrediting organizations. Nevertheless, as students within a school of public health, they will be exposed to ways of thinking and problem-solving, and concepts that take them beyond the confines of their specific disciplines, allowing them to see and understand the individual within the context of the health of the community. Thus the school of public health gives these students a new set of lenses through which to view reality and to develop a greater appreciation for community-based lifelong learning. At the same time, public health professionals will have available potential "laboratories" for the application of public health principles.

Consider, as an example, the discipline of speech-language pathology. These practitioners provide services in a variety of organizational settings, such as schools, hospitals, nursing homes, and home care agencies. Traditionally speech-language pathologists have been educated within schools of education. However, approximately 50 percent of them will practice within a health care setting; those practicing within schools will treat children whose health conditions or disabilities warrant care by practitioners who are more "medically" knowledgeable.

Speech-language pathologists provide services to children and adults from diverse demographic and socioeconomic backgrounds. Their education within a school of public health will enhance their ability to see the individual patient or client within the context of personal and social characteristics that greatly impact their lives and their response to treatment, and their sensitivity to situations that warrant further investigation from a public health perspective. Furthermore, to the extent that speech-language pathologists are exposed to public health competencies, they will bring to the front line of health care organizations (including, in some cases, the patient's home) and community schools an additional source of public health education.

Collaboration with other disciplines not only strengthens students from other professions but brings to schools of public health new ideas and concepts, contributing to the transdisciplinary approach to education.

TRANSDISCIPLINARY RESEARCH

Public health research differs from biomedical research in that its focus is on the health of groups, communities, and populations. Rather than focusing on the mechanism of disease at the cellular or organ system level, it focuses on the origins of disease as it relates to human activity— in human behavior, interactions with the environment, and within societies. Prevention of injury and disease and their control within defined populations—not treatment of individuals—is the intended application for the knowledge public health research yields. Public health research answers the questions: What are the consequences to human health of the way we live, and what can be done to improve it? As discussed previously, the committee views this approach within the framework of the ecological model of public health.

Many changes in the scope and conduct of such research during the coming century can already be anticipated and will be briefly outlined here. What is unlikely to change is the reality that schools of public health will serve as the nidus for much if not most of that research. Some health agencies (e.g., the Centers for Disease Control and Prevention [CDC] and state departments of health) and other organizations in the private sector (e.g., industry and pharmaceutical companies) will continue to sponsor and conduct public health research. However, the academic community and, in particular, schools of public health will likely continue to carry the major responsibility for public health research.

The most striking change in public health research in the coming decades is the transition from research dominated by single disciplines, or a small number, to transdisciplinary research. *Transdisciplinary research* involves broadly constituted teams of researchers that work across disciplines in the development of the research questions to be addressed. Traditionally, research has been either interdisciplinary or multidisciplinary in nature. Interdisciplinary refers to the collaboration of two investigators from different departments or fields to answer a question of joint or mutual importance. An example might be an urologist and an epidemiologist participating in a study to find a new cause of bladder cancer. Multidisciplinary refers to research that offers the potential to resolve questions of both mutual and separate interest among participating investigators. For example, the urologist and epidemiologist identified above might be joined by an industrial hygienist interested in developing a new model for measuring coal tar pitch volatiles. Likewise, a cancer biologist might want to use the study to test the value of a new immunologic tool for early cancer detection. While the output of his/her work would be used by the epidemiologist, separate research questions would pertain to the additional disciplines.

Transdisciplinary research implies the conception of research questions that transcend the individual departments or specialized knowledge bases, typically because they are intended to solve applied public health research questions that are, by definition, beyond the purview of the individual disciplines. In transdisciplinary research broadly consituted teams of researchers work across disciplines in the development of the nature of the public health problem to be resolved. For example, the "team" might now include an economist, health psychologist, and chemical engineer to compare alternative strategies for reducing bladder cancer risk including development of a pitch substitute, economic incentives to eliminate pitch, or methods to cajole all exposed subjects to come early and often for screening.

In the current paradigm, the prominent research mode is for single disciplines to join in interdisciplinary or multidisciplinary research. Research methodology typically reflects the repertoire of the principal investigator's discipline, complemented by consultant co-investigators with additional skills. For example, at present a chronic disease epidemiologist might study the effect of an ambient air pollutant on mortality. He would obtain input from an environmental chemist to help measure the independent variable (air pollutants) and a biostatistician to allow exploration of advanced causal models. By definition, transdisciplinary research goes beyond and transcends individual disciplines by crossing traditional professional boundaries; individuals strive to adapt their own discipline's theories and research to the needs of other disciplinary members of the group—each is able to transcend his individual perspective. The practical ramifications of such an approach are that the disciplines will no longer function like "silos" that exist side-by-side, deeply rooted in their respective traditions. Rather, these disciplines will involve more broadly constituted and integrated "teams."

For example, study of the health impact of air pollutants could involve more broadly constituted "teams" comprised of social scientists (to measure covariation in health status caused by social factors that in the present paradigm would be viewed as "confounders"), experts in lung and cardiovascular biology (to evaluate early markers of health effect because mortality, while easily measured, is too crude an end-point given the broad and diverse population at risk), and perhaps industrial engineers and economists to evaluate, in the research context, the feasibility and costs associated with alternative strategies for modifying air quality.

Another example of the transdisciplinary approach is demonstrated by considering the prevalent public health concern, diabetes. Diabetes is especially prevalent among minority populations of American Indians, African Americans, and Hispanics. Lifestyle in terms of diet, weight, and lack of exercise can be contributing factors. Moreover, the availability of services, be they medical services including physician awareness for screening, or the availability of healthy food alternatives, are environmental factors that add complexity to individual lifestyle choices.

Further, service patterns are determined in part by demographics, for example, the urban and rural nature of place, the ethnic and racial make-up of community, and the relative degree of affluence or poverty. Cultural patterns also are expressed in the types of food that groups eat and the traditions and attitudes that groups hold toward medical interventions. Furthermore, policy has an impact on the attention devoted to diabetes, for instance, how much funding is dedicated to research, prevention, and treatment.

When the public health researcher is confronted by diabetes, an ecological framework is most pertinent because the disease has complex and interacting components that are individual behavioral and psychosocial, community, cultural, social, economic, and political as well as biological. Inter- and multidisciplinary models, in which disciplines share input, are valuable but do not blend the perspectives to produce a holistic view of the problem and possible research solutions.

The practical ramifications of the transdisciplinary approach to education are that schools of public health may need to rethink their structure and modes of instruction in order to develop professionals that can interact synergistically when confronting health concerns. Fundamental questions arise when moving toward a transdisciplinary educational focus, such as does it make sense, in this day and age, to retain single discipline courses and departments that reinforce singular specialties by educating in the traditional silos. Perhaps it makes greater sense to structure education with a blending of disciplines by concentrating on public health case studies such as diabetes, so that comprehensive public health responses are melded in the educational process itself. A transdisciplinary approach that emphasizes the ecological model for addressing complex health issues may well result in more effective interventions.

Closely related to the move toward more transdisciplinary approaches to complex health issues such as the one discussed above will be the move toward more *intervention oriented* research. In most domains of biomedical investigation, research regarding the mechanism of a disease is followed by study of therapeutic interventions, resulting in new strategies for disease diagnosis or treatment. In public health the linkage between discovery of etiology and strategies for control and prevention has not followed a biomedical research pathway, because the link is fundamentally social. Recognition of causal factors contributes to improvements in public health only insofar as feasible, socially palatable, and economically viable intervention strategies can be established. As such, rigorous testing and evaluation of interventions will increasingly dominate the landscape of public health research and will most likely become a dominant theme distinguishing public health from other aspects of biomedical research.

Not surprisingly, the study of interventions will, in turn, dictate the third sea-change in public health research: *community participation*. Whereas the study of clinical interventions can usually be achieved by recruiting consenting patients or subjects, interventions at the community level require an altogether different paradigm, in which investigators and the community or population to be studied are partners. Models for such research already exist (see discussion in Chapter 3). However, the preeminence of such research in schools of public health in the coming decades will mandate new expertise in these research modalities. In addition, such research will fundamentally alter relationships between schools of public health, the communities in which they are embedded, and the public and private agencies with responsibility for the health of these communities or populations.

The committee recommends that schools of public health reevaluate their research portfolios as plans are developed for curricular and faculty reform. To foster the envisioned transdiciplinary research, schools of public health may need to establish new relationships with other health science schools, community organizations, health agencies, and groups within their region.

Schools of public health have a primary responsibility for educating faculty, researchers, and senior-level practice professionals. The challenges of the 21st century require an educational approach that is ecological in nature, an approach that emphasizes the determinants of health and their interaction. Education for public health in the 21st century requires cultural competence, and broad new competencies in information technology, communication, and genomics, and a vast reemphasis on practical aspects of training.

POLICY

The Future of Public Health aptly characterized public health as a "problem-solving activity" and described the "appropriate and fundamental" role of politics in health policy-making (IOM, 1988). Public health professionals across the disciplines of public health cannot be fully effective without an understanding of how policies are made and put into practice (Burris, 1997; Gostin et al., 1999; Gebbie and Hwang, 2000; Reutter and Williamson, 2000; Weed and Mink, 2002). An ecological understanding of public health only makes this skill set more salient. Identifying social determinants of health means challenging settled practices, institutional arrangements, and beliefs that are perceived to be beneficial to at least some members of the community.

Schools of public health play a primary, albeit variable, role in health policy development and dissemination. In addition, the application of policy, which by nature includes understanding the politics of policy development and implementation, must be addressed. Simply put, using the crude formula that "science + politics = policy," dwelling on the science without appropriate attention to both politics and policy will not be sufficient for schools to be significant players in the future of public health and health care. The appreciation of the importance of this role and the more systematic incorporation of policy efforts being linked to the schools' educational mission are critical to charting the future. These same elements must also be enriched in research and service missions of schools of public health.

Academic public health leaders—whether they reside in schools of public health, public health programs, medical schools or elsewhere—are often turned to for information needed in the formulation of policy. They are viewed as credible spokespersons who can make issues understandable to decision makers, the media, and the public. Faculty researchers are contributing greatly to the rapidly growing new knowledge about critical health care challenges, such as the multiple determinants of population health, the effectiveness and quality of health care delivery, and environmental hazards and their control. Yet the very same experts are at worst steered away from and at best not encouraged to move along the continuum from science to policy. Even if induced to do so, most faculty are not prepared to do so effectively, nor are faculty colleagues available to assist them. Part of the disincentive for researchers is that the current academic reward system generally acknowledges only research productivity and not the translation of scientific findings and knowledge to inform evidence-based policy making. This must change if schools are to maintain, let alone enhance, their status as important players in the public health and health care delivery arena.

The committee believes that it is the responsibility of schools of public health to better prepare their graduates to understand, study, and participate in policy related activities. Therefore, **the committee recommends that schools of public health:**

- **enhance faculty involvement in policy development and implementation for relevant issues;**
- **provide increased academic recognition and reward for policy-related activities;**
- **play a leadership role in public policy discussions about the future of the U.S. health care system, including its relation to population health;**
- **enhance dissemination of scientific findings and knowledge to broad audiences, including encouraging the translation of these findings into policy recommendations and implementation; and**
- **actively engage with other parts of the academic enterprise that participate in policy activities.**

ACADEMIC COLLABORATION

The events of fall 2001 made it evident that public health systems need to have strong collaborative relationships with all parts of the health system, and all health professionals need to have a solid grasp of public health principles and practices. Community-based physicians and hospital-based nurses were rapidly involved in surveillance and public education (and in some cases administration of prophylaxis). Community members turned to their neighborhood health centers and providers for assistance in interpreting media reports and defining levels of risk. In many cases, those from whom help was sought were themselves seeking to understand who was in charge, how the public's health was being protected, and what information was reliable. One way to strengthen the capacity to respond is to increase the proportion of health and related professionals who have had a solid introduction to public health as a part of their basic professional education.

Some other schools have existing requirements for public health, community health, or preventive medicine content but may not see these as central to their mission and thus may not give them sufficient attention. In other cases, the public health content may not be required, but would enhance the ability of the graduate to be an active part of a community health system. It is not the responsibility of a school of public health to solve the curricular problems of other schools or to monitor the education provided there. In fact, assumption of such roles would not be met with pleasure from the other schools. The expertise of a school of public health, however, in public health sciences, the ecological approach to health, or in specific topics such as risk communication or community partnerships could be useful to faculty in other schools.

At some level, the relationship of a school of public health with other health-related schools and departments could be seen as parallel to the relationship between a local health department and other health-related resources in the community. Following that model, public health experts can make themselves available partners in defining educational goals for public health units or courses, in developing classroom or other teaching resources, and in looking for opportunities to allow students from multiple disciplines to work with public health students in models consistent with a 21st century view of improving the public's health.

Therefore, **the committee recommends that schools of public health actively seek opportunities for collaboration in education, research, and faculty development with other academic schools and departments, to increase the number of graduates in health and related disciplines who have had an introduction to public health content and interdisciplinary practice, and to foster research across disciplines.**

ACCESS TO LIFE-LONG LEARNING

Earlier in this chapter we asserted that schools of public health should focus on preparing senior-level public health professionals, leaders, researchers, and faculty. This is a primary role for schools of public health. However, a secondary, but essential role of schools of public health as well as of other public health education programs is to provide continuing education to the existing workforce in two different ways. The first is new training reflecting evolutions in the field in order to update skills. The second is to provide the basic education needed by workers who have no previous training in the public health aspects of their positions.

Because of the breadth and depth of their expertise across all disciplines of public health and their regional and national presence and influence, schools of public health have a responsibility to *assure* that appropriate, high quality education and training are available to the current and future public health workforce. In fulfilling this assurance role, schools contribute to enhancing the professionalism of public health. Schools are not, however, the sole direct providers of such training. The assurance role, often accomplished by working with partners in the community, is analogous to that of the public health system which does not always provide the necessary health services to individuals or communities but assures that their health care needs are met.

There are several models that might be considered for assuring that education and training of the current and future public health workforce are available. An uncommon model, but one frequently believed to be predominant, is one in which schools of public health assume the sole responsibility for this comprehensive education and training. Under this model, schools, in addition to preparing graduate-level public health practitioners, provide training for current public health employees who may or may not have had any public health training through a variety of educational modalities. While there are some schools of public health that fulfill this role, it is not the norm for the majority of schools, nor do we envision that it should be.

Schools of public health do, however, have a role to play in providing education and training to the larger workforce, given their enormous expertise in the various disciplines of public health that underlie public health practice. Additionally, faculty are experienced in developing, presenting, and evaluating educational material, in assessing student learning, and in using various pedagogical modalities. Distance learning provides one mechanism through which these strengths are increasingly being used for training and continuing education of the public health workforce. Recent technological developments have made the expertise of school faculty potentially more accessible to many public health agencies and organizations that are not located near schools of public health.

Unfortunately, not all health departments have the necessary technological capabilities to take advantage of distant training opportunities. In addition, the transmission of knowledge in certain public health disciplines is not easily accomplished through distance learning. Furthermore, some public health workers desire education and training in a classroom setting. For situations in which distance learning is not feasible or desirable, schools of public health should partner with local educational institutions. Many locales throughout the nation have community colleges or other two-year institutions. Schools of public health, through partnerships with these institutions, can provide the educational materials and instructor support for localized public health training. This also will give students in alternative settings the opportunity for exposure to public health courses and public health careers.

Finally, it is recognized that basic public health training related directly to practice is often better provided by the local and state health departments than by schools of public health. However, schools of public health have a critical role in assisting health agencies in the development of training materials, providing expertise in the delivery, presentation, and evaluation of the materials, and in the assessment of student learning. For example, through the University of Washington Northwest Center for Public Health Practice, a network of state and local health departments in Alaska, Idaho, Montana, Oregon, Washington, and Wyoming, has been established with funding from CDC and the Health Resources and Service Administration (HRSA). The network will assess public health workforce training and preparedness needs and develop appropriate materials, including materials for distance learning, for use by various educational institutions in these states.

Schools of public health are well positioned, because of their institutionally neutral location, to coordinate the sharing of "best practices" across public health agencies and the development of information networks among the agencies. For example, faculty members with expertise in environmental health could develop and maintain a Web site for the exchange of important information relevant to state environmental health directors.

Schools of public health also provide more individualized education and training on specialized topics to the public health workforce. A faculty member from environmental health with particular expertise on assays for different types of microbes found in water could, for example, be available to respond to queries. State public health laboratories and local health directors could request information about the appropriate assays or, if local facilities are not available, the expert could conduct the assay in his or her lab. Local health department directors frequently consult with academic epidemiologists about protocols for responding to infectious disease or food-borne outbreaks.

There are many potential roles that schools of public health have, either directly or indirectly, in the education and training of the public health workforce. Depending on the mission, expertise, resources, funding, and capacity of any particular school, it may do all or only a selection of the above. However, the broad knowledge and expertise of schools of public health in public health disciplines and educational methodology positions them well to assure that comprehensive, high quality public health workforce education and training is available in the region served by each school. Therefore, **the committee recommends that schools of public health fulfill their responsibility for assuring access to life long learning opportunities for several disparate groups including:**

- **public health professionals;**
- **other members of the public health workforce; and**
- **other health professionals who participate in public health activities.**

COMMUNITY COLLABORATION

The previous sections have focused on the responsibility of schools of public health as they relate to practitioners, researchers, and educators within the field. However, there is a much larger audience with which schools of public health are inextricably linked; that audience is the public and the communities within. Implementing effective interventions to improve the health of communities will increasingly require community understanding, involvement, and collaboration. Schools of public health have a responsibility to work with communities to educate them about what it takes to be healthy and to learn from them how to improve public health interventions.

Through research and service, schools of public health have the opportunity to engage communities in the task of improving the health of the public. The report, *New Horizons in Health* (IOM, 2001b) describes the importance of increased research funding for the study of communities. For schools of public health, the commitment to community must incorporate and emphasize community-based research, but also address the other key missions of teaching and service, including policy development and advocacy, as discussed earlier.

Schools of public health will play a leadership role in advancing knowledge about the multiple determinants of health and how to apply this knowledge in varied arenas, including governmental policies and programs. The research base for much of this knowledge and the application of the knowledge will largely be community-based. Traditionally, single or multiple investigators have considered the community a "laboratory," in much the same way that clinical investigations viewed the bedside as the laboratory. But the future calls for a different approach, one recognizing that by collaborating with the community (geographically or otherwise defined), both schools of public health and the community will benefit. Community organizations and leaders must have the opportunity to contribute to and influence research (often research on intervention effectiveness) that has the potential to address local needs. Schools of public health can direct their expertise to generating and analyzing appropriate local level data and targeting significant problems. By working with the community, students in schools of public health will be exposed to far more coherent and visible community-based learning experiences.

Schools of public health will be most effective in engaging in new relationships with their communities if they take a leadership role in collaborating with other important academic units, for example, medicine, nursing, education, urban planning, and public policy. Given the premise of a future where the boundaries of medicine and public health continue to blur, and the recognition that protecting and promoting population health requires consideration of a broad array of non-biological factors, schools of public health would be well served to not go down this path alone.

Therefore, **the committee recommends that schools of public health should:**

- **position themselves as active participants in community-based research, learning, and service;**
- **collaborate with other academic units (e.g., medicine, nursing, education, and urban planning) to provide transdisciplinary approaches to active community involvement to improve population health; and**
- **provide students with didactic and practical training in community-based public health activities, including policy development and implementation.**

Further, community-based organizations should have enhanced presence in schools' advisory, planning, and teaching activities.

FACULTIES FOR SCHOOLS OF PUBLIC HEALTH

The curricular changes envisioned by the previous discussion will likely require substantial changes in the composition and backgrounds of future faculties of schools of public health. As schools of medicine have discovered, especially the "research intensive" schools, faculties most adept at careers in peer-reviewed and funded biomedical research, whether in basic science departments or clinical departments, are neither sufficient nor entirely satisfactory to meet the demand for educating medical students and post-graduate trainees in the practice of medicine. Accordingly, most have developed separate faculty tracks for "clinician-educators"—faculty whose primary role is classroom and bedside teaching, roles increasingly incompatible with the demands of success in the laboratory or even in patient-focused research. In a similar fashion, faculties for schools of public health in the future will require both research-oriented and practice-focused components.

A major barrier to increasing emphasis on practice and service relates to faculty rewards, promotion, and tenure because, within academic institutions, public health practice is not valued as highly as research activity nor is it rewarded by most academic institutions. Developing a system and criteria for evaluating the scholarly contributions of practice activities is imperative. Maurana and colleagues (2000) propose four standards for assessing the scholarly contributions of practice and service activities: (1) the service must have significance in that the issues addressed are of importance and value to project goals; (2) the context of the service is crucial in that it should have a close fit with the environment, should utilize appropriate expertise and methods, should have a substantial degree of collaboration, and should sufficiently and creatively use resources; (3) the scholarship of the service should demonstrate appropriate application, generation, and use of knowledge; and (4) the service should be able to demonstrate impact to issues, institutions, and individuals.

A second model, the Competency-Based Model of Alverno College in Milwaukee, Wisconsin, divides scholarly activity into four competencies, each of which specify skills, activities and requirements that faculty must master in order for promotion. Further, the Association of Schools of Public Health (ASPH, 1999) asserts that

> *service is relevant as scholarship if it requires the use of professional knowledge, or general knowledge that results from one's role as a faculty member. This knowledge is applied as consultant, professional expert or technical advisor to the university community, the public health practice community or professional practice organizations. The dimension of scholarship distinguishes practice-based service from a form of service known traditionally as the general responsibilities of citizenship.*

For faculties with the appropriate mix of backgrounds and skills to be recruited and sustained, **the committee recommends a major change in the criteria used to hire and promote school of public health faculty. Criteria should reward experiential excellence in the classroom and practical training of practitioners.** One approach might be to place greater emphasis on public health *practice* research and service activities. Another approach may be to develop academic tracks based on teaching and practice. If this approach is taken, such tracks need to be sufficiently comparable to the existing tracks to encourage the choice of a teaching career in public health among professionals with these orientations, and sufficiently attractive to ensure heavy demand for the posts from among the best potential candidates.

As detailed in Chapter 2, the funding stream historically has fostered emphasis within schools of public health on the research function. Such an imbalance has impeded maximizing the contributions of schools in practice and education. Moreover, the traditional single-discipline approach to agency funding has limited the repertoire of public health research. Recommendations to correct problems associated with funding have been proffered in Chapter 6 of this report. The committee emphasizes that it believes research, practice, and teaching are all important, both to the future of schools of public health and to the health of the populations served by graduates of those institutions.

As discussed in Chapter 2, funding for public health education has risen and fallen over the course of the 20th century. Currently, funding for health education programs and schools of public health remains problematic, making it difficult for schools of public health as well as other programs to institute the necessary changes recommended by this report. **The committee acknowledges the major contributions of philanthropic foundations to the development of public health education in the United States and emphasizes the renewed importance of foundation support to fund new initiatives and experiments in public health education.** However, greater support for public health education is needed from state and federal governments to ensure that a competent, well-educated public health workforce is available (see Chapter 6 for specific recommendations).

Public health professionals, knowledgeable about the ecological approach to health and educated in a transdisciplinary fashion, are essential to preserving and improving the health of the public. Well-educated researchers are needed to help us understand the kinds of interventions and policies that lead to improved health and the kinds of barriers that must be overcome to design and implement effective interventions. Knowledgeable faculty, with both practice experience and research expertise, are needed to prepare the next generation of practitioners and researchers with necessary competencies. Highly trained practitioners are needed for leadership and senior positions of responsibility to guide the development and implementation of programs, policies, and systems that will benefit the health of the public. Schools of public health are uniquely positioned to educate these professionals but can only do so if sufficient funding is available to develop the programs and approaches necessary to prepare future public health professionals for the challenges and opportunities of the 21st century. Recommendations for such funding are discussed in Chapter 6.

The following chapter discusses the role of programs and other schools in educating public health professionals.

5

The Need for Public Health Education in Other Programs and Schools

In addition to schools of public health, other programs, schools, and institutions play major roles in educating public health professionals. The committee believes that to provide a coherent approach to educating public health professionals for the 21st century, it is important to examine and understand the potential contributions these other institutions and programs can make. Therefore, this chapter will discuss graduate programs in public health, schools of medicine, schools of nursing, and other professional schools.

GRADUATE PROGRAMS IN PUBLIC HEALTH

As discussed in Chapter 2, a significant number of new entrants to the field of public health and existing public health workers receive their masters of public health (M.P.H.) education and training in graduate programs in public health. In contrast to "stand alone" schools of public health in university settings, these programs are generally housed within other academic departments (such as departments of preventive medicine in schools of medicine), colleges, or schools in university settings such as education. In fact, these M.P.H. degree-granting graduate programs appear to be growing at a faster pace than schools of public health although the number of students per program tends to be smaller than the number per school.

The Council on Education for Public Health (CEPH) accredits not only the schools but also graduate programs in Community Health Education (CHE) and in Community Health/Preventive Medicine (CHPM), while the Accrediting Commission on Education for Health Services Administration (ACEHSA) accredits programs in health administration. CHEs offer degrees solely in health education; whereas CHPMs may offer a variety of concentrations, and presently tend to be heavily weighted toward epidemiology, health administration, environmental health, maternal and child health, and general public health.

In the 1970s, some of these programs sought an umbrella under which they could loosely federate for purposes not dissimilar to the role played by the Association of Schools of Public Health for schools. Because many of these early programs were housed in medical school departments of preventive medicine, it was not surprising that they sought a home base through the Association of Teachers of Preventive Medicine (ATPM) rather than create their own organizational structure. Thus, within ATPM, the Council of Graduate Programs in Public Health and Preventive Medicine, as it is now known, came into being.

In 1999, ATPM's Council, with collaboration from CEPH, surveyed the CHE, CHPM, and other M.P.H. programs to collect data on students, graduates, faculty, areas of concentration, etc., based on the 1998–1999 academic year. Results of the survey indicated that there were 75 programs in existence at the time, although others were in some phase of planning a program. The breakdown of the 75 programs surveyed indicated their accreditation status as:

Accredited	38
Pre-accredited	4
Application for accreditation	9
Not accredited	24

Some of the respondent characteristics and findings indicated that about two-thirds of the students were attending part-time. The programs are generating about one in every eight M.P.H. degrees, are practice oriented, and tend to be located in states lacking schools of public health (although the Tufts University program co-habits in the Boston area with schools of public health at Harvard and Boston Universities). For some programs this is a transition phase to becoming a school but a significant number, especially CHEs, will remain programs.

According to Bialek and Bialek (1999), during the 1990s significant changes were made in some public health education programs, including increased emphasis on cross-disciplinary education and use of problem-solving and case-based approaches to learning. These programs are contributing significantly to the formal graduate-degree-granting educational process for leadership in the future public health workforce and for continuing education opportunities in the existing workforce at all levels. When this reality is combined with the potential for housing educational programs within major state and local health departments and collaborating with undergraduate institutions, the importance of these programs to the education of public health professionals is further highlighted. The committee recognizes the contributions to the education of public health professionals that have been made by these programs and encourages programs to make further advancements in public health education. Therefore, **the committee recommends that these graduate M.P.H. programs in public health institute curricular changes that:**

- **emphasize the importance and centrality of the ecological model, and**
- **address the eight critical areas of informatics, genomics, communication, cultural competence, community-based participatory research, global health, policy and law, and public health ethics.**

MEDICAL SCHOOLS

Physicians have historically played a central, though not exclusive, role in ensuring the health of the public. The Hippocratic physicians knew the importance of the physical and social environment to the health of communities:

> *Who ever wishes to investigate medicine properly should proceed thus: in the first place to consider the seasons of the year, and what effect each then produces. Then the winds . . . in the same manner, when one comes into a city to which he is a stranger, he should consider the situation, how it lies as to the wind and the rising of the sun . . . one should consider most attentively the water . . . and the mode in which the inhabitants live, and what are their pursuits, whether they are fond of drinking to excess, and given to indolence, or are fond of exercising and labor (Hippocrates, 400 B.C.).*

In the late 19th and early 20th centuries, most public health professionals were physicians (Hager, 1999) who contributed greatly to public health. During the 19th century, the physician John Snow conducted a series of classic epidemiologic studies of the cholera epidemic in London in 1854. During the early 20th century, William Gorgas, a physician working with the U.S. Army Corps of Engineers, implemented an extensive program of mosquito eradication in the Panama Canal Zone and virtually eliminated yellow fever among workers on the canal (McCoullough, 1978). A. Bradford Hill, a biostatistician who later became a physician, explored the relationship between cigarette smoking and lung cancer along with his colleague Richard Doll, providing the first strong empirical evidence of the association between smoking and cancer.

Beginning in the 20th century, however, the association between public health and mainstream medicine declined (although many physicians continue to lead or participate in local, state, and national public health efforts). In fact, increasing tensions resulted in a schism between medicine and public health. Reasons for this tension include the following:

• Public health was viewed as infringing on the doctor-patient relationship when it called for reporting communicable diseases.
• Public health agency delivery of health care services was viewed as economically threatening to the medical profession.
• The rise of the tertiary care hospital furthered separation.
• Basic views of promoting health widely differed, with medicine focused on individual care and the biomedical paradigm while public health focused on prevention (Brandt and Kass, 1999).

Table 5-1, lists traditional distinctions between medicine and public health, identified by Fineberg, that contribute to our understanding of why this separation has occurred. In 1950 about 30 percent of graduates of public health education programs were physicians. By 1988 that figure had shrunk to 22 percent of graduates, and half of these were from countries other than the United States (Bialek and Bialek, 1999).

However, meeting the public health challenges of the 21st century will require that medical, scientific, and public health communities work together. Reasons include the changing spectrum of health problems and the crisis in health care costs (Lasker, 2001), development of scientific and methodological underpinnings of medicine and public health (Tuckson, 1999), and the slowly changing values of purchasers and the growth of generalism and primary care (Shine, 1999). The divergence between medicine and public health that developed in the 20th century must be corrected because, in the words of Koplan and Fleming (2000), the two fields "share in the responsibility and have an unprecedented opportunity to apply current knowledge to improve the health of the nation." An adequate infrastructure and joint training and research opportunities should be created to support a productive collaboration of medicine and public health. Advances in genetics and bioinformatics create a unique opportunity for these two fields to join forces in preventive care of chronic diseases, susceptibility to which can now be detected decades earlier.

There have been previous efforts to bridge the chasm between medicine and public health. The 1998 conference Education for More Synergistic Practice of Medicine and Public Health (sponsored by the Josiah Macy, Jr., Foundation) was organized to discuss the most effective ways to "educate and train physicians and public health professionals to collaborate more effectively" (Hager, 1999). During that conference, Lasker (1999) urged that medical students learn the relevance of population-based methodologies and population-based strategies to the provision of medical care. The conference concluded that the "spirit of collaboration" must

TABLE 5-1   Traditional Distinctions Between Medicine and Public Health

Medicine	Public Health
Primary focus on individual	Primary focus on population
Personal service ethic, conditioned by awareness of social responsibilities	Public service ethic, tempered by concerns for the individual
Emphasis on diagnosis and treatment, care	Emphasis on prevention, health promotion for the whole patient and for the whole community
Medical paradigm places predominant emphasis on medical care	Public health paradigm employs a spectrum of interventions aimed at the environment, human behavior and lifestyle, and medical care
Well-established profession with sharp public image	Multiple professional identities with diffuse public image
Uniform system for certifying specialists beyond professional medical degree	Variable certification of specialists beyond professional public health degree
Lines of specialization organized, for example, by: • organ system (cardiology) • patient group (pediatrics) • etiology, pathophysiology (oncology, infectious disease) • technical skill (radiology)	Lines of specialization organized, for example, by: • analytical method (epidemiology) • setting and population (occupational health) • substantive health problem (nutrition)
Biological sciences central, stimulated by needs of patients; move between laboratory and bedside	Biological sciences central, stimulated by major threats to health of populations; move between laboratory and field
Numeric sciences increasing in prominence, though still a relatively minor part of training	Numeric sciences an essential feature of analysis and training
Social sciences tend to be an elective part of medical education	Social sciences an integral part of public health education
Clinical sciences an essential part of professional training	Clinical sciences peripheral to professional training

SOURCE: Permission to print from author, Harvey V. Fineberg, M.D.

diffuse through both medicine and public health, with students in the fields of medicine and public health needing exposure to the academic disciplines and practice of the other.

Current changes in the delivery system also foster the need for physicians educated in basic public health. The number of physicians working in settings such as a health maintenance organization (HMO) or a large multidisciplinary group is increasing; academic physicians also work in large health systems. These systems must account for the overall health of a group of patients. With a growth in the numbers and the size of systems has come increasing demand for physicians to play a more central role in planning the delivery of health care to patients in these systems. Further, physicians have become much more aware (as have other health care professionals) of the impact of population health upon individual practice. Examples include the threat of bioterrorism, medical care cost constraints that require developing priorities, and the rising interest in health promotion and disease prevention among the population at large.

Because of these changes, it is important that schools of medicine incorporate into their core curriculum basic public health education such as

- basic screening techniques for adverse health habits (such as smoking and alcohol/drug abuse);
- nonpharmacological preventive strategies (such as smoking cessation and weight reduction);
- the costs and benefits of various screening methods (such as mammography and PSA screening for prostate cancer); and
- population monitoring of disease burden (such as tracking both acute and long lasting epidemics).

Because medical school curricula are already tightly organized, it may appear difficult to introduce another area for learning. The first two years of medical school are spent on basic science preparation which is followed by clerkships in clinical disciplines during the third year. The fourth year features a mixture of elective and required course work in disciplines such as radiology, anesthesiology, and the medical and surgical subspecialties (Anderson, 1999). However a growing number of medical schools include social science in the required curriculum and provide opportunities for work with other health care professionals. In 1998 it was reported that 56 of the 125 accredited U.S. medical schools taught separate required courses on such topics as public health, epidemiology, and biostatistics and that 36 medical schools offered a combined M.D. (doctor of medicine) and M.P.H. degree (Anderson, 1999).

There are existing examples that, with some modification, could produce professionals with both an M.D. and either an M.P.H. or Ph.D. (doctoral) degree in public health. Graduates of these programs would have the requisite education to become leaders to bridge the chasm between the two disciplines. In the joint program linking the University of California at San Francisco (UC San Francisco) and the school of public health at the University of California at Berkeley (UC Berkeley), for example, 12 students are admitted by a joint admissions committee from the UC San Francisco School of Medicine and the UC Berkeley School of Public Health. They spend the first three years at Berkeley, during which they satisfy the preclinical requirements of medical school and complete a thesis for a master's (M.S.) degree in public health from Berkeley. They then transfer to UC San Francisco to complete the third and fourth years of medical school and graduate with the M.D. degree from UC San Francisco.

The joint program linking Duke University and the University of North Carolina is organized somewhat differently. Between 20 and 25 students out of 100 third-year medical students at Duke elect to enroll at the University of North Carolina School of Public Health. In addition to a generic M.P.H. degree developed for physicians interested in public health, students work toward degrees in epidemiology, maternal and child health, health services administration, or environmental health sciences. Given Duke's unique curriculum (which permits a year of scholarship during the four years of medical school), students who elect this program can acquire an M.P.H. and an M.D. degree within four years.

The program at the University of Southern California is an example in which the Keck School of Medicine and the Master of Public Health Program (located within the medical school) work together. Students from the school of medicine can insert a year between their second and third years of medical school to complete the M.P.H. degree in the public health program, returning to the medical school to complete their M.D. degree training.

The committee's goal in developing recommendations for programs and approaches for public health education in medical schools is to foster improved public health training for *all* medical students. We envision a future in which one-fourth to one-half of medical school graduates are fully trained in the ecological model of health at the M.P.H. level. An ecological understanding of health and a transdisciplinary approach require physicians who are fully prepared to work with others to improve health. Therefore, **the committee strongly recommends that:**

- **all medical students receive** *basic* **public health training in the population-based prevention approaches to health;**
- **serious efforts be undertaken by academic health centers to provide joint classes and clinical training in public health and medicine; and**
- **a significant proportion of medical school graduates should be** *fully* **trained in the ecological approach to public health at the M.P.H. level.**

Further, when a school of public health is not available to collaborate in teaching the ecological approach to medical students, the committee recommends that medical schools should partner with accredited programs in public health to provide for public health education.

Medical schools and schools of public health should collaborate on educational and scientific programs that address some of our most prevalent and troublesome chronic diseases, such as Alzheimer's disease, obesity, and severe or unremitting psychiatric disorders. Evidence of the success of such collaboration can be found in the area of cardiovascular diseases and, to some extent, various cancers. Additionally, ongoing collaborations between schools of medicine and public health could focus on understanding how recent advances in genomics and biomedicine in general will make an impact on the public's health over time. Students in both schools should be exposed to dialogues between leaders in medicine and leaders in public health on central topics related to the public's health (e.g., regarding the impact upon and cost to society of new generation, subject specific pharmaceutical products).

Therefore, **schools of medicine and schools of public health should develop an infrastructure to support research collaborations linking public health and medicine in the prevention and care of chronic diseases.**

SCHOOLS OF NURSING

Nurses constitute the single largest group of professionals practicing public health. The estimated numbers available are somewhat inconsistent, given various data sources and definitions. In the 2000 estimated enumeration of the public health workforce, nearly 11 percent of the professionals identified were nurses, and there are probably a good many more practicing under more general job titles. (Center for Health Policy, 2000) These data come primarily from state and local health departments. However, many additional nurses in public health practice are employed elsewhere, including departments of education, as school nurses; workplaces, as occupational health nurses; community clinics, as educators and outreach coordinators; hospitals, as epidemiologists; and in voluntary health organizations in a wide range of population-focused activities. In most local public health departments, nurses are the largest component of the workforce. In very small departments they may be the only health professional staff member(s) (Gerzoff et al., 1999; Richardson et al., 2001). Anecdotal information suggests that states moving to establish local public health agencies or offices have made nursing the first locally based office, often using federal grant or reimbursement mechanisms for funding.

The complexities of the field of nursing are illustrated in the fact that leadership for public health nursing and public health nursing education comes from a multi-organizational group known as the Quad Council of Public Health Nursing Organizations. Members include the Association of State and Territorial Directors of Nursing, the Association of Community Health Nurse Educators (ACHNE), the Public Health Nursing Section of the American Public Health Association, and the American Nursing Association (ANA). Regular communication within the Quad Council has meant that the interests of the practice field are regularly brought to the attention of educational institutions and, concomitantly, that the educators are in a position to share emerging insights in education and research with practice leaders. Key documents on public health nursing, such as the statement on scope and standards of community health nursing practice (QCPHNO, 1999) published by the ANA, are developed with the full collaboration of this entire group. The state nursing directors are also in a position to share emerging concerns of the public health nursing community with the broader public health practice field through their organizational relationship as an affiliate of the Association of State and Territorial Health Officials.

Confusion regarding the roles of nurses in public health practice and education has been fostered by a decades-long debate about terminology: community health nursing as identical with or different from public health nursing. The distinction may be an important one: the mere fact that one is working in an office, a van, or on a street corner may not signify that one is concerned about the health of groups or populations, or focused on prevention. For example, the increasing use of home health and visiting nurses has meant that more and more nurses are providing individual clinical nursing care in patients' homes rather than in hospitals. These nurses may not, however, be paying attention to family dynamics, environmental health, or health education and promotion as included in public health nursing practice since the days of Lillian Wald, who first coined the term (Erickson, 1987; Byrd, 1995). Given shifts in approaches to medical care, it is appropriate that nurses learn how to provide clinical services in a wide range of settings, including homes and community sites. This does not, however, replace the role that nurses have played and should continue to play on interdisciplinary public health teams working to improve the health of communities through disease prevention and health promotion. The two require different education and developmental opportunities, though a well-prepared public health nurse may provide clinical services as a response to community need or as a way of supporting a position that also has a community focus.

As is also true for physicians, all nurses are at some level a part of the public health system, given their potential contributions to the control of nosocomial infections, the identification of conditions of public health importance, and the education of patients and families about disease prevention and health promotion. These roles may be more visible in some specialty areas (e.g., the role of nurses in obstetrical units in promoting child health) or some settings (outpatient departments in underserved rural and inner city communities), and may or may not be explicitly recognized in job descriptions or in the work of the local official public health agency. However, because of their important contributions, it is important that all nurses have at least an introductory grasp of the role of public health in the community and of the principles of health promotion and disease prevention and, as discussed below, the curriculum standards for schools of nursing support this concept.

Undergraduate Education

Since early in the 20th century, the stated standard of preparation for a public health nurse has been the baccalaureate degree (AACN, 1999). This requirement was based on an understanding that working in the community required knowledge of community and family dynamics beyond that necessary for effective practice within an institutional setting. As standards for baccalaureate nursing education were established, public health nursing was included as a required classroom and clinical experience, and this can be seen as the major distinguishing clinical feature that differentiates the baccalaureate level of nursing education from diploma or associate degree programs. The ANA has created Standards for Public Health Nursing Practice (QCPHNO, 1999) that provide the standards against which practice should be measured. The licensing board in at least one state (California) continues to issue a separate certification for public health nursing and limits use of the title "public health nurse" to those who are so certified. The exact content of these public health nursing courses has changed over time, as have the associated clinical experiences.

Guidelines for nursing education are provided through the school accreditation process and through standards set by educators in various specialty areas. Accreditation of schools can be done by one of two organizations, the National League for Nursing Accrediting Commission, Inc., or the American Association of Colleges of Nursing (AACN). The AACN only accredits programs at the baccalaureate or higher level and includes the expected competencies items such as social justice, community health risk assessment, health promotion, risk reduction and disease prevention, human diversity, and global health care, all of which are basic for good public health practice.

Standards for associate degree programs (and the dwindling number of hospital-based diploma programs) are established by the National League for Nursing Accrediting Commission, Inc., the accrediting body. At the associate degree level, the standard requires that the curriculum provides for attainment of knowledge and skill sets in community concepts, health care delivery, critical thinking, communications, therapeutic interventions, and current trends in health care.

There is nothing in the standard that suggests that these graduates are being prepared for the level of analytic skills and community dynamics that are a key part of public health nursing practice. Because of job market pressure, however, many health departments recruit and hire graduates of associate degree programs (especially in communities in which there is no baccalaureate school of nursing), and the schools are responsive to inclusion of material that might make their graduates even more employable. Informal discussions would indicate that an increasing number of schools at this level are including community-based clinical practice within the curriculum but not classic population-focused public health nursing.

Additional guidance on public health nursing is provided by the Association of Community Health Nursing Educators. This group contributed to the development of the ANA scope and standards, and has produced guidance on the content of public health nursing education at the undergraduate and graduate levels. Members are primarily faculty from baccalaureate and master's degree nursing programs. There is no organizational link to any group representing more general public health professional education, such as the Association of Teachers of Preventive Medicine. A continuing concern of faculty in schools of nursing is identification of appropriate sites for clinical experience. As public health agencies have been caught up in the provision of clinical services, it has been easier to provide students with home health or other non-institutional personal care experiences and more difficult to provide community-focused experiences. As agencies operate programs with ever-tighter budgets and staffing patterns, they may also be reluctant to accommodate student space and time needs, meaning that even those students graduating from programs listing public or community health in the curriculum may have had minimal experience in population-focused practice.

Graduate Education

Nurses interested in advancing their skills in public health nursing practice may pursue education in public health at a school of public health, earning the master of public health degree. While at one time there were more, today only one school of public health continues to offer an M.P.H. program specific to public health nursing. Alternatively, some schools of nursing offer masters-level programs in public health or in community health nursing. Classically, these programs emphasize community assessment, development of programs of health promotion and disease prevention, use of public health analytic skills, and application of nursing knowledge and skill in the community setting. These programs have become smaller, and many have closed, as schools of nursing have concentrated master's level preparation on midwives, nurse anesthetists, nurse practitioners, and other advanced practice nurses. Some of these advanced practice nurses are in specialty areas closely related to public health programs (midwifery, pediatric or family nurse practice). The National Organization of Nurse Practitioner Faculty (NONPF) has had philanthropic support for the last three years to encourage the inclusion of public health and population-focused concepts in the advanced practice nursing curricula (Community Health Resource Center, 2000). These graduates will not be fully prepared in public health analytic or community development skills; their exposure is intended to prepare them to better work as partners with patients and communities (such as in community-based primary care programs). While any of these programs based in schools of nursing may provide excellent courses and theoretical programs, it is only with great difficulty that students are provided with opportunities to explore the interdisciplinary nature of public health practice during the learning period.

Graduate education in public health or in nursing is held to be the standard for nurses moving to supervisory or leadership positions in public health organizations. The uneven geographic distribution of education programs and the location of many public health organizations in rural and underserved areas means that not all practicing nurses can easily attain this desired higher education before moving up a career ladder. Current discussions in nursing education circles emphasize the need for graduate nursing programs to extend themselves via distance learning opportunities and collaboration with practice sites to facilitate advanced learning, without the necessity of leaving job and family for extended periods (Wedeking, 2001). The Health Resources and Services Administration (HRSA) has funded a number of projects that involve collaboration across schools of nursing and practice organizations to support such a commitment. One example is the project funded through the University of Illinois-Chicago School of Nursing Peoria campus, linking multiple nursing schools with health departments and other employers of public health nurses to strengthen the curriculum, increase the number of masters degree graduates, and recruit additional nurses into public health, particularly those from ethnic or racial minorities. Another program housed at the University of Colorado is linked with the University of Wyoming and with health departments in both states, providing access to graduate education through distance learning across the region.

Nursing Education and the Job Market

While the standard for public health nursing practice is the baccalaureate degree, with the master's degree preferred for leadership positions, the realities of the nursing education and job market are such that many agencies will undoubtedly continue to fill positions with under-prepared nurses rather than leave them vacant. The problems are exacerbated by the continuing nursing shortage in both the public health and the health care systems. Half of all practicing nurses are educated at the associate or diploma level, and there is little likelihood that this will shift in the near future. In some geographic areas, the only source of nursing education is the local community college. The increasing competition with hospitals for the aging nursing workforce means that slower-moving public employers are unable to compete regarding salary and benefits with other systems. To the extent that public health nurses are employed in other than public settings, they may benefit from this competition. It is extremely difficult to require graduate education for those in nursing leadership positions because of the competition with other organizations to fill positions. Too often public health organizations are struggling to fill nursing vacancies before the funding for the position evaporates. Lack of adequate funding resources also affects the nurse who has gained public health knowledge through on-the-job experience, has moved to a nursing supervisory or management position, and might well be ready for a broader public health program leadership position. Lacking a formal educational credential, these nurses find themselves blocked from advancement. Because many nurses are place-bound by family obligations, they will not be able to move forward until either nursing or public health graduate education is more readily available.

Continuing Role for Schools of Nursing

The roles for nurses in public health practice in public health agencies, community-based practices, and elsewhere is such that the long-standing identification of the baccalaureate degree as the entry to public health practice is likely to remain the standard, even though it is often honored in the breach. Undergraduate schools of nursing will continue to be a major source of entry-level public health workers. **The committee recommends that these undergraduate schools be encouraged to assure that curricula are designed to develop an understanding of the ecological model of health and core competencies in population-focused practice.** Because of the ongoing debate about preparation of the associate degree graduates in community skills, **the public health community should offer assistance in identifying the appropriate level and type of position for these graduates as well.** In support of sound baccalaureate-level preparation in public health nursing, **the public health community should be attentive to the need for student clinical experience, should collaborate in making appropriate sites available, and should consider ways to assure that nursing education does not occur in a vacuum apart from the full range of professionals practicing in public health.** One approach to collaboration would be development, by schools of public health, of "liftable" public health curricular modules that could be shared with other institutions as they develop courses aimed at providing education in public health.

The graduate-level role for schools of nursing is not so clear. The inclusion of public health perspectives and skills in clinical programs in a range of specialties as advocated by NONPF supports the appropriate orientation of clinicians to their roles in collaboration with public health. With the exception of employment as clinicians in specific program areas, however, these are not the nurses to which public health will be looking for leadership. **Schools of nursing that offer master's degree programs in public health nursing should be encouraged to partner with schools of public health to assure that current thinking about public health is integrated into the nursing curricula content, and to facilitate development of interdisciplinary skills and capacities.** Programs offering joint degrees in nursing and public health that bring the two schools together formally offer a viable and effective option for advancing public health nursing practice.

OTHER SCHOOLS

An ecological theory of health suggests that health emerges from the day-to-day interactions between people and their environment. A population's health reflects how it does business, what it does in its spare time, how it is housed, the organization of its cities, its way of solving problems, and its distribution of wealth and status (Link and Phelan, 1995; Marmot, 2000). In this view, health issues arise everywhere that people make and implement decisions about how to organize and carry on daily life. Health is a consequence (and too often an unrecognized consequence) of the activities and decisions of a wide range of social actors for whom health is not mentioned in their job descriptions. Both as citizens in a democracy and as participants in the creation of the conditions of social life, the responsibility for health rests upon each of us.

Public health is, by most prevailing definitions, a collective enterprise. It is what we do together as a society to attain the conditions in which we achieve the widest distribution of the highest level of health we can manage (Gostin et al., 1999; IOM, 1988). Yet, as has been repeatedly observed, securing public support for public health work can be difficult (IOM, 1988); indeed, public health issues often seem "invisible" in policy debates (Burris, 1997). Americans often see matters of health in individualistic, medical terms. Yet as Geoffrey Rose long ago made clear, many important questions of health must be asked and answered in terms of population-level causes and effects (Rose, 1985). Given the centrality of health in all of our lives, and the complexity of organizing collectively in a democracy to achieve it, there is a strong case to be made that curricula at all levels should include more training on health and human ecology. "Health literacy" can and should be a goal of our educational system as a whole (St. Leger, 2001).

More specifically, the committee believes that the diffusion of health issues and responsibilities in society creates a need for health training in a range of jobs without health in the title. The enterprise of public health cannot succeed as a niche speciality. Creating the conditions in which Americans can be healthy requires the informed collaboration of planners, executives, and lawyers. Indeed, there are many professions whose practitioners play an important role in health, and whose trainees are appropriate candidates for health training.

Law plays essential roles in public health. As a tool for regulation, it provides incentives for healthy behavior and deters insalubrious activities (Gostin, 2000). It structures and limits public health activities (Burris, 1994; Gostin et al., 1999). Laws and regulations provide public health with various powers under certain conditions, ranging from the authority to quarantine individuals through civil and criminal enforcement when necessary to protec the health of citizens. More fundamentally, an ecological view of health reveals the role of law in structuring social determinants of health, in mediating their effects, and as a tool of "structural intervention" at the level of policy (Blankenship, 2000; Burris et al., 2002).

Public health is marginal or entirely missing as a component of the curriculum at most of the country's nearly 200 law schools (Goodman et al., 2002). Without training in public health, it is not surprising that lawyers in practice—as advocates, legislators, executives, and judges—have difficulties unraveling complex health issues. As Parmet and Robbins observe, "thinking like a lawyer" does not currently include adopting a public health perspective. Cases are brought, decisions are made, and statutes are drafted with a profound effect upon the public health, yet with little appreciation of what that means. Thus, the U.S. Supreme Court in *Bragdon* v. *Abbott* seemed confused about what it means for the Centers for Disease Control and Prevention to be unable to prove that seven dental workers who were HIV-positive had not been exposed at work. The dissent went further, suggesting that risks can be assessed without considering denominators. Likewise, the Supreme Court rejected state regulation of tobacco marketing, failing in a fundamental way to comprehend that public health is not a matter of individual choice (Parmet and Robbins, 2002).

Renewed appreciation of the importance of socio-economic factors in public health points to business as a neglected but crucial actor in public health (Woodward and Kawachi, 2000). From the availability of HIV/AIDS drugs (James, 1998) to the prevalence of fast-food outlets (Nestle and Jacobson, 2000), the conditions of health reflect decisions by national and international concerns. Business decision-makers, moreover, are community leaders. Their partnership is recognized as essential in developing and implementing collective health strategies (Williams et al., 1991; Sumartojo, 2000). Setting aside the question of regulation, the importance of business to health suggests the value of training future business leaders about the health consequences of their decisions. Like other activities, business can be informed by ethical considerations (Danis and Sepinwall,

2002), which, in turn, depend upon a grasp of the underlying facts about how economic factors influence health. However, the practice of public health can benefit from better understanding and use of business management techniques (Guarino, 1997).

Urban planning—including zoning, design, sanitary regulations and construction standards—was one of the most pressing preoccupations of 19th century public health (Duffy, 1990; Novak, 1996). During the 20th century, the health aspects of planning grew less pressing, and the focus of the profession turned elsewhere. While the proposition that planning matters to health would not be disputed in the urban planning profession, health concerns remain on the periphery of training and practice. Yet as new research continues to show, the physical environment matters to health (Cohen et al., 2000), and planning can be a tool of intervention—or a means through which social inequalities produce health inequalities (Bullard and Johnson, 2000; Maantay, 2001).

The committee believes that public health is an essential part of the training of citizens, and that it is immediately pertinent to a number of professions. Specialized interdisciplinary training programs, such as those offering joint J.D. and M.P.H. degrees or joint M.P.H. and M.U.P. (masters of urban planning) degrees can create specialists and are important. Our view, however, is that more is needed. Public health literacy, entailing a recognition and basic understanding of how health is shaped by the social and physical environment, is an appropriate and worthy social goal. Further, education directed at improving health literacy at the undergraduate level could also serve to introduce persons to possible careers in public health. **The committee recommends that all undergraduates should have access to education in public health.**

It is beyond both our charge and our capacity to make specific recommendations about how to incorporate health into diverse curricula. Doubtless the usual challenges to curricular change will arise—faculty flexibility, scarce resources of time, and student interest. **The committee does, however, stress the importance and recommend the integration of a more accurate and ecologically oriented view of health into primary, secondary, and post-secondary education in the United States.**

This chapter has emphasized the importance of public health education in graduate programs of public health and in other schools and institutions of learning. The following chapter examines the role of local, state, and federal agencies in educating public health professionals.

6

Public Health Agencies: Their Roles in Educating Public Health Professionals

The previous two chapters have reviewed the role of schools of public health and of other programs and schools in educating public health professionals. While the committee is aware that public health professionals work in a variety of settings, there is a special relationship with the governmental public health agencies at the local, state, and federal level. These agencies have a major responsibility for educating and training the current public health workforce and future public health workers who have not received training elsewhere.

The following sections discuss activities and roles of local, state, and federal public health agencies. These discussions are followed by a series of recommendations targeted at what official public health agencies can do toward better educating public health professionals.

LOCAL PUBLIC HEALTH AGENCIES

Activities and Responsibilities

Local health departments (LHDs) have a fundamental and complex role as the front line for delivery of basic public health services to most of the communities in this country. There are nearly 3,000 local health departments in the United States, varying dramatically in geographic size, size and nature of population, urban and rural mix, economic circumstances, governmental structure within which they work, and governing organization to which they are accountable. The majority of local health departments provide a wide variety of services to very diverse communities with limited resources and too few staff (the median size is 14 full-time equivalents). Although local public health services are often discussed within the framework of the 10 Essential Public Health Services, the services actually provided vary widely from state to state, from urban to rural areas, and are especially adapted to address local priorities and concerns. Despite considerable variation, however, more than two-thirds of local health departments provide the following core services: adult and childhood immunizations; communicable disease control; community outreach and education; epidemiology and surveillance; environmental health regulation such as food safety services and restaurant inspections; and tuberculosis testing (NACCHO, 2001).

The past decade has been a period of significant challenges and transitions in local public health. For many LHDs, resources for some traditional services have been shrinking at the same time that challenges and demands have been increasing. More people lack health insurance and are looking to "safety net" providers for health care. Rapidly growing immigrant communities are creating a need for new services or for providing traditional services in a different way. Many LHDs are shifting from "personal health care" services to "population-based" services. In the aftermath of bioterrorism, health departments have greatly increased disease surveillance activities and are now at the center of many of the federal, state, and local emergency planning activities. With these challenges and changing circumstances, there is increasing urgency for an assessment of how new public health professionals are educated and how the current workforce can be trained for new skills. The education and training of the public health workers poses a difficult challenge to local health departments, one for which they will require the engagement and support of many partners, most notably the schools that educate health and public health professionals.

Training and Education in Local Health Departments

LHDs have serious and urgent needs for preparing new public health professionals and for upgrading the skills of current public health professionals (NACCHO, 2001). They face an on-going need to train new and current workforces in how to respond to emerging areas, changing diseases, new priorities, and new technologies. Because LHDs are experiencing significant changes in the types of services they provide and the roles they are expected to fulfill, education and training are needed to prepare new and current local public health staff to meet these changing expectations.

As discussed earlier, the vast majority of current public health workers do not have formal public health training. Many have training in a primary health profession, such as nursing or environmental health, and continue to receive training updates from the schools and through their professional associations. One of the major training needs for LHDs is the capacity to support their professional staff in maintaining their professional credentials or licensure through on-going continuing education. Much of the training for local public health staff is obtained through the initiative of individual employees, seeking continuing education in areas of special interest to them or for the continuing medical education or continuing education units that are required to maintain their professional credentials.

LHDs provide a significant amount of direct staff training, primarily for focused technical skills specific to their services and programs. Most LHDs have very limited financial and staff resources for providing or obtaining training or for supporting education for their staff, and they rarely have staff who are professionally prepared to be trainers or educators. Linkages with schools of public health could enhance the capacity of LHDs to provide broader and higher quality training.

LHDs can play an important role in training and education by assessing the skills and training needs of their workforce. This assessment role is proposed in the National Public Health Performance Standards (NPHPS) (CDC, 1998), as part of Essential Service 8 (Assure a Competent Public and Personal Health Care Workforce) (Public Health Functions Steering Committee, 1994). The NPHPS also proposes that LHDs adopt "continuous quality improvement and life-long learning programs for all members of the public health workforce, including opportunities for formal and informal public health leadership development." They further recommend that LHDs "[p]rovide opportunities for all personnel to develop core public health competencies."

Many sources of education and training are currently available for local health department staff, including state government agencies, professional organizations, academic institutions, federal government agencies, consultants, other local government agencies, and in-house training (Bialek, 2001). However, there is little systematic information about the extent to which LHDs actually use various sources, which courses and topics are most frequently sought, or the effectiveness of the alternative sources of training. "Distance learning" has become increasingly available, but there has been no assessment of the level of use or value for local public health professionals.

Incentives for Public Health Training for LHD Professionals

Most LHD professionals do not have formal public health training. Few M.P.H. graduates work in LHDs, at least in part because pay scales of LHDs usually are not competitive. Also, most LHDs are unable to provide support or incentives for current staff to obtain the formal public health training that would increase the quality of the workforce. For example, they have limited ability to provide tuition reimbursement or educational leave to current employees who might wish to obtain an M.P.H. Most LHDs cannot provide pay increases or other incentives to staff who obtain additional public health training or degrees.

The National Public Health Performance Standards recommend that LHDs "[p]rovide incentives (e.g., improvements in pay scale, release time, and tuition reimbursement) for the public health workforce to pursue education and training (Essential Service 8). This will become possible only if additional resources become available to LHDs. In many cases, significant changes would also be required in local government personnel rules and systems. Efforts should be directed toward engendering increased understanding and financial support from local governments as well as from other funders and policy makers, regarding the importance of on-going training and a higher level of initial education for staff working in public health.

LHDs as Partners with Programs and Schools of Public Health

Partnerships linking LHDs with programs and schools of public health would offer many potential benefits to both partners. The National Public Health Performance Standards recommends that LHDs "[p]rovide opportunities for public health workforce members, faculty and student interaction to mutually enrich practice-academic settings" (Essential Service 8).

Field Placements

Field placement programs are probably the most frequent collaborative activity that currently occurs between local health departments and academic institutions for health professions. Most of the students are at the baccalaureate level. Students participating in field placement programs rarely or never receive financial support from either the academic institution or the health department. The student field experience varies widely among the programs and schools of public health. Implementation of this committee's recommendations related to improving the practice experiences of students in schools of public health (see Chapter 4) would greatly enhance the value of these experiences for both the students and LHDs.

Staff and Faculty Exchanges

Local health department staff offer practical experience that could be of value in the education of public health and other health professionals.

Available information suggests that staff and faculty exchanges are not currently a major collaborative activity between local health departments and academic institutions for health professions. LHD staff and academic faculty might benefit substantially from programs allowing them to spend significant time in such activities. Many LHDs have indicated that they would be interested in having department staff placed in faculty appointments (Bialek, 2001). Such interest corresponds well with the committee recommendation (see Chapter 4) that there be enhanced participation of practitioners in the education of students in schools of public health. Other activities offering the potential for collaboration include special projects, seminar courses in the academic setting, and practical training in LHDs. Few LHD staff serve on academic institution steering or advisory committees.

Research Opportunities

Because LHDs are intimately involved with their communities, they have an immediate and detailed knowledge about local public health issues that need to be investigated. They also have the types of credibility with those communities that would facilitate community-based research, providing another cornerstone for working collaboratively with faculty and the community to facilitate such research.

Local Public Health Leadership

Because persons in leadership positions in LHDs are responsible for setting the policies and priorities of their departments and also for coaching and training their subordinate staff, it would be desirable for these leaders to have formal education in the full range of public health principles and skills. However, a 1992–1993 survey of LHDs showed that 78 percent of LHD executives had no formal public health training, although executives of larger jurisdictions were more likely to have a public health degree (NACCHO, 2001). Many LHD leaders do not have access to the financial support nor the educational leave necessary to obtain a formal public health degree. Flexible and creative approaches, such as certificate programs and public health leadership institutes, are needed to provide substantial public health training to the majority of the current LHD leadership.

The many state, regional, and national public health leadership institutes that have arisen in recent years are of increasing prominence as sources of training for these upper-level LHD professionals. The leadership institutes are important sources of training in management and leadership skills for the current workforce. In some cases, they also provide training in public health theory to current managers who do not have formal public health training. Many of these leadership institutes are linked with or located within academic institutions, in some cases schools of public health.

Many different organizations and professions contribute to the health of a community, but local governmental public health agencies have a special, fundamental role. They provide services that either cannot be provided or will not be provided by anyone else. In most cases, local health departments provide the most basic public health services in a community, while also establishing the framework for the network of population-based services provided in the community. As we write this report, local health departments are increasingly engaged in emergency and bioterrorism preparedness. A decade ago, LHDs faced the emerging epidemic of AIDS and HIV. To respond effectively to the current and to future challenges, LHD professionals need the ability and resources to rethink and refocus services and to adapt as each new problem arises, as the population changes, or as the community expectations evolve. To do this effectively, they need an ecological perspective and preparation that is grounded in the fundamental skills of public health.

Local public health officials welcome the diffusion of public health approaches and methods of analysis and approach into other components of the health services system and related fields. At the same time, there is a striking disconnect between the current focus of the academic institutions for the public health profession and persons actually practicing in the field. This results from a very complex set of demands and constraints, discussed earlier, including the limited funding available to provide meaningful practice experiences in both education and research. Although this quandary is not easily resolved, it must be confronted and addressed to ensure that the future leaders of state and local public health will have the professional skills and knowledge that they require to effectively address our public health needs.

Local public health works closely with community health care providers, and all health professionals should function to some degree as part of their community's system of public health. Therefore, public health at the local level would be greatly enhanced by including basic public health education in the training of all health professionals. It would be a great benefit to our public health services and to our communities if all physicians, nurses, and other health professionals had some education in basic public health concepts and systems. In particular, they need familiarity with legal context and responsibilities, the meaning and value of a "population health" approach, and epidemiologic techniques. This improves their ability to work appropriately with their local public health department. Associations representing LHDs have participated in national discussions urging that education of all health professionals should be competency-based and should recognize the broad determinants of health, including social determinants.

STATE PUBLIC HEALTH AGENCIES

The 1988 Institute of Medicine report *The Future of Public Health* described the need for well-trained public health professionals who can address the needs of the public health system associated with technological advances, leadership and political will, and social justice. That report briefly described major barriers to meeting those needs: lack of public health training among the leadership of public health systems, lack of financial resources, and the general limitations of the governmental environment. Those observations were significant for the times, but that landmark report did not offer additional analysis regarding the issue of workforce development. Much has changed during the past decade and a half. Since 1989, new challenges for public health have emerged, with new emphases on surveillance of complex disease patterns and syndromes, emergency preparedness with regard to chemical and biological terrorism, and the increasing diversity of the population as a whole. These challenges have escalated at a time when most states are dealing with budget cuts, personnel hiring freezes, and difficulty in recruiting and hiring public health professionals. Since two-thirds to three-fourths of the state health departments' budgets are personnel related, the cost of weak workforce development is magnified.

The Organizational Climate

All states and territories and the District of Columbia have a designated entity known formally as the state public health department. There are a total of 56 such designated units in the United States and its territories. The mission, authority, governance, and accountability of these agencies vary according to the state statutes that establish the public health departments. Some are located within a comprehensive health and human services umbrella agency; some are divisions within the governor's organizational structure; and some are stand-alone state agencies. According to the Association of State and Territorial Health Officials (ASTHO), in 2001, 35 state health departments described themselves as free-standing agencies, while 21 listed themselves as being part of a larger umbrella agency.

The executive-level leadership of state health departments also varies. Most states have statutory requirements for the appointment of the state health official, but the legal requirements differ. Twenty-eight states require the official state health executive to hold a license to practice medicine in the state; others do not. The state health department's organizational climate will often emulate the philosophy of the top executive, especially with regard to workforce development. Therefore, the educational background and previous experience of the state health official is important to the process of educating the public health workforce.

Regarding the mission of the organization, the majority of state public health departments have published mission statement language that describes protecting and promoting the health of the public. Most states have a combination of state and local health departments; some states operate the local health departments; and a few states have no local health departments at all.

State level public health staffs are often health professionals without public health degrees. Regarding governance, 34 state public health agencies have a state level board of health, while 22 state public health agencies do not. Seven state public health departments are designated as the official environmental health agency. Four state public health departments are the official mental health agency. Four state public health departments are the official Medicaid agency.

Recent emphasis on the development of state-level public health system performance measures offers an exceptional opportunity to articulate the unique role of state health departments within the overall public health system. The process of developing measures has challenged ASTHO, the Centers for Disease control and Prevention (CDC) and other partner organizations to delineate the basic public health functions that all states have in common, regardless of variations in organizational structures. Based on the set of essential public health services (see Box 6-1), performance measures enable states to take an enterprise-level view of key functions that must be in place to improve population-based health. The 10 Essential Public Health Services, by their nature, cut across categorical distinctions and allow for a more universal perspective on the principal state public health capacities and functions. The state health department's role in any given state is to facilitate the implementation of the Essential Public Health Services, either by carrying them out directly or by indirectly supporting the efforts of the local public health agencies, and to articulate the needs of the public health workforce to federal partners.

Responsibility of the State Health Department

One of the 10 Essential Public Health Services specifically focuses on assuring a competent public health and personal care workforce, and state health departments have specific responsibilities in this area. Continuous improvement in the quality of services delivered to the citizens of a state includes an ongoing and systematic assessment of the profes-

---

BOX 6-1 Essential Public Health Services

Assessment
1. Monitor health status to identify community health problems
2. Diagnose and investigate health problems and health hazards in the community

Policy Development
3. Inform, educate, and empower people about health issues
4. Mobilize community partnerships to identify and solve health problems
5. Develop policies and plans that support individual and community health efforts

Assurance
6. Enforce laws and regulations that protect health and ensure safety
7. Link people to needed personal health services and assure the provision of health care when otherwise unavailable
8. Assure a competent public health and personal health care workforce
9. Evaluate effectiveness, accessibility, and quality of personal and population-based health services

Serving All Functions
10. Research for new insights and innovative solutions to health problems

---

SOURCE: Public Health Functions Steering Committee, 1994.

---

sional workforce available to deliver those services. The following sections describe specific components of a state-based public health system quality review process related to workforce development.

Review of the Public Health System's Progress Toward Achieving Goals and Objectives from *Healthy People 2010*

For the first time, these national health objectives also contain a call to improve the public health infrastructure. Specifically, states are encouraged to address the need for workforce development in areas related to public health competencies, and continuing education regarding the 10 Essential Public Health Services. States are challenged to develop specific, measurable strategies for action. States who use the *Healthy People 2010* objectives to measure their progress must deal with the subject in a direct, measurable way.

Concern for Deterioration in 2002 of State Fiscal Conditions, as Nearly Every State Reported a Budget Gap to Their Legislature

The National Conference of State Legislatures (NCSL, 2001) conducted a survey to ascertain the extent of the problem. Results of the survey revealed that although most of the problem relates to revenue shortfalls, many states are now facing spending overruns. Unfortunately, the Medicaid shortfalls have occurred at the same time that many states have also experienced budget shortfalls in public education and corrections. Therefore, most state programs, including public health departments, have been affected by these budget constraints. Fifteen states and the District of Columbia have earmarked reserve funds to get through this fiscal year, and another 10 states are considering doing so. Eight states have plans to use their tobacco settlement funds, not for expansion programs or services, but to support the current budget. Other budget management issues have included shifting financing for previously approved projects to cover the budget shortfall in other areas; instituting hiring freezes; redirecting special fund revenues into the general fund; boosting gaming revenues; delaying scheduled tax cuts and increasing state employee contributions to health care plans. The net effect is that, at the very least, public health departments will not have stable funding for improving population health and may in fact, lose critical resources. Despite competing demands and insufficient resources, states are attempting to conduct detailed reviews of human and capital resources as well as trying to provide public health services. Workforce development programs often are the first to be eliminated when state budget constraints emerge. State health departments have a pivotal role in assuring that the workforce available in these difficult times is well trained and well prepared to fulfill its important functions. The leadership of the state health departments is critical to assuring this objective.

Continuum of Workforce Development Assessment Activity Should Exist in States Where Personal Health Service Delivery Remains a Viable Activity

Some states use interdisciplinary teams comprised of nurses, social workers, nutritionists, and clerical staff to conduct reviews of the patient care process through the use of standardized tools, often developed by the team. Clinical indicators for program areas might also be considered in reviews of this nature as means for determining whether a more detailed review is required. Environmental health program components, if applicable, are typically included in this type of review. For example, a program for reducing lead poisoning should include an assessment of environmental exposure to lead-based paint or other sources, and methods to abate this exposure. The underlying strategy for this level of review is a focus on process of care or the delivery of specific services. State health departments have the responsibility for assuring that standards are in place for conducting these reviews, and for policies and procedures that provide for the continuing learning needs of staff. Continuing learning needs may also have to address the natural tension that exists for those staff that have responsibility for assuring both personal and population-based health.

Program Staff at the State Level of a Public Health Agency Might Work with Their Respective Local Staff to Review County or Regional Progress Toward a Program's Overall Goals and Objectives

Items included in this type of review process are generally categorical in nature and may include target population information, status reports on progress toward health status changes, and comparisons with other geographical entities. Review may include process, impact, and outcome components. Full program evaluations may also be conducted on a regular basis, using models that vary from state to state. In many states, the tools used to review program status are developed or adapted by state level program staff, with technical assistance or input from federal program staff or local public health staff. State-level public health program directors and consultants need to work in an organizational environment that provides them with the tools to manage their programs and to provide leadership to local public health agencies in that regard. Assurance of this type of learning environment requires an ongoing commitment to assessing the needs of this sector of the public health workforce and partnering with programs and schools of public health to develop programs to meet those needs.

Window of Opportunity

The recent appropriation of federal dollars for emergency preparedness provides a potential window of opportunity for state health departments to make much-needed progress in workforce development. Appropriation of the money through the existing cooperative agreements with the CDC requires that a portion of the emergency preparedness plans address workforce development and education. At the time of this writing, the plans were under review. However, it appears many states will use the opportunity provided by this funding to develop strong relationships with schools of public health for the assessment of public health workforce needs and the planning of multiple strategies to meet those needs. Opportunities to enhance the distance learning technology within states also have been provided, using a variety of methods. State health departments would be wise to use this time of resource availability to conduct their own training readiness inventory in order to foster organizational climates that favor strong workforce development programs. One method for assessing a state's readiness to provide leadership in the development of the public health workforce is through the use of the National Public Health Performance Standards (CDC, 1998).

National Public Health Performance Standards Program

The role of state health departments in assuring a competent public and personal health care workforce has been described in the National Public Health Performance Standards Program, Essential Service 8 (ensuring a competent public health and personal health care work force) which identifies the responsibilities of state public health departments as including the education, training, development, and assessment of health professionals—including partners, volunteers, and other lay community health workers—to meet statewide needs for public and personal health services. Responsibilities also include the development of processes for credentialing technical and professional health personnel, the adoption of continuous quality improvement and life-long learning programs, and the development of partnerships with professional workforce development programs to assure relevant learning experiences for all participants. Continuing education in management, cultural competence, and leadership development programs are also responsibilities of the state public health agency.

The National Public Health Performance Standards identify indicators of success for a state public health agency to utilize in evaluating whether it is meeting the workforce development needs of its jurisdiction. Indicators of success include the following:

• Identification of the workforce providing population-based and personal health services in public and private settings across the state and implementation of recruitment and retention policies. This indicator includes an assessment of the number, qualifications, and geographic distribution of the public health workforce statewide.

• Provision of training and continuing education to assure that the workforce will effectively deliver the Essential Public Health Services. These plans involve resource development programs that include training in leadership and management, multiple determinants of health, information technology growth and development, and support of competencies in the specific health professions. The state public health agency should be instrumental in assuring that these functions are conducted, regardless of whether the agency provides the functions directly or facilitates their provision.

• Provision of specific assistance, capacity building, and resources to local public health systems in their efforts to assure a competent public and personal care workforce. This indicator includes the collaborative development of retention and performance-improvement strategies to fill workforce gaps and decrease performance deficiencies; and assurance of educational course work to enhance the skills of the workforce of local public health systems. State public health agencies, working in collaboration with local public health systems, can develop incentives that support workforce development activities.

• Evaluation and quality improvement of the statewide system for workforce development. To be successful in this area, the state public health agency would periodically and consistently review the state's activities to assure that a competent public and personal care workforce uses the results from reviews to improve the quality and outcome of its efforts. These reviews would include current and future workforce distribution and continuing education needs as well as public health system assessment for its success in meeting those needs.

The public health system in the United States has been described as being ill-prepared, in disarray, and under-funded to meet the current (much less the future) needs of the population (IOM, 1988). Attention is being paid to the development of multiple strategies to strengthen the public health infrastructure. If these strategies are to be successful in the future, the developmental and educational needs of the public health workforce must be addressed. If the historic underfunding of public health human resource development continues, the public health system as a whole will be further weakened. State public health agencies, working in partnership with local public health systems and the federal government, must take the lead in strengthening the quality of the public health workforce.

FEDERAL PUBLIC HEALTH AGENCIES

Federal agencies are important to the development of the public health workforce generally, and specifically to the education of public health professionals. The roles of these agencies have included developing the research base that provides education; testing educational approaches; helping schools develop infrastructure; supporting faculty development; and providing funding for students. Key agencies include the National Institutes of Health (NIH), the Health Resources and Services Administration (HRSA), CDC, the Substance Abuse and Mental Health Services Administration (SAMHSA), and the Agency for Healthcare Research and Quality (AHRQ), and their predecessors. They are located within the Department of Health and Human Services (DHHS), but the size of the department and the diversity of missions of the component units makes it critical that the discussion be specific to the individual agency.

From the broadest public health education perspective, HRSA and CDC have been central and will be the focus of this discussion. HRSA includes the Bureau of Health Professions (BHPr), which has the mission to help to assure access to quality health care professionals in all geographic areas and to all segments of society. BHPr puts new research findings into practice, encourages health professionals to serve individuals and communities where the need is greatest, and promotes cultural and ethnic diversity within the health professions workforce. The bureau identifies several specific programs for the public health workforce:

• Public Health Training Centers assess workforce learning needs and provide tailored distance learning and related educational programs.
• Public Health Special Projects community and academic partnerships improve skills and competencies of the public health workforce, provide distance learning, curriculum revision, and course content in areas of emerging importance.
• Public Health Traineeships train eligible individuals in public health professions experiencing critical shortages.
• Preventive Medicine Residencies support existing and develop new residency training programs, and provide financial assistance to enrollees.
• Health Administration Traineeships and Special Projects increase the number of underrepresented minority health administrators and the number of health administrators in underserved areas, support academic and practice linkages, and develop outcomes-based curricula.

Beyond these programs, other HRSA components that focused on maternal and child health, HIV/AIDS, primary care, and rural and migrant health have included support for preparation of workers to attend to issues that are both personal care and public health in nature. The most recent visible activity of HRSA in public health workforce development has been the funding of 14 Centers for Public Health Training, supporting school of public health-based efforts to strengthen ties between practice and academics, offer improved distance-based continuing education, and work toward a stronger, more diverse public health workforce.

The CDC's predecessor agencies were the source of early efforts to identify the public health workforce and encourage the development of public health agencies in local jurisdictions across the nation. The programs of CDC have supported technical training for public health laboratory staff and for program staff in tuberculosis control, sexually transmitted disease control, HIV/AIDS prevention, school health, and, more recently, in chronic disease prevention and injury prevention. The Public Health Practice Program Office has provided a home base for the multi-organization Public Health Workforce Collaborative, begun in partnership with HRSA and involving nearly every identifiable organization representing some segment of public health workforce development. An Office of Workforce Planning and Policy (OWPP) was created as the organizational locus for external workforce development activities within CDC and the Agency for Toxic Substances and Disease Registry (ATSDR) (a recommendation of the CDC/ATSDR Strategic Plan for Public Health Workforce Development, 2000). The OWPP assures coordination and accountability for implementing the strategic plan, oversees the development of workforce policies and standards, and convenes partners, as needed, to address issues and to provide support and technical assistance. The goal is to improve the ability of public health workers, nation-wide, to perform the essential services of public health, and to prepare the workforce to respond to current and emerging health threats.

The CDC has funded 15 Centers for Public Health Preparedness based in schools of public health that are specifically charged to assure that the nation's public health workforce is ready to respond to emergencies, especially those associated with bioterrorism. This specialized activity has eclipsed the more general support for implementing the Strategic Plan for the Development of the Public Health Workforce created in 2000.

The potential roles for federal agencies in developing the public health workforce for the 21st century could take several forms, and are in the following categories:

- Research
- Development of academic programs
- Development of faculty
- Support for students
- Continuing education
- Technology development
- Modeling

Research

The education of public health professionals is built on a very slender research base. There is little or no research to support advancing the M.P.H. degree as the hallmark of readiness to practice public health, or on the differential contributions to public health of persons educated in various combinations of professional and on-the-job programs. Neither is there a research base on the relationship of staff preparation to outcomes of public health programs. While there has been discussion of building a public health systems research base (parallel to that available for studying questions about personal care and the medical care system), only the first steps have been taken. The federal agencies, especially CDC and HRSA, should make funds available for this important research, either as specifically funded studies or as components of other research portfolios.

Development of Academic Programs

Federal agencies should continue to support schools of public health and other institutions that train public health professionals (e.g., schools of nursing, medicine, dentistry, environmental sciences, and others), especially by providing pilot funds for the development of curriculum in emerging areas of practice (e.g., the eight content areas of informatics, genomics, communication, cultural competence, community-based participatory research, policy and law, global health, and public health ethics that were identified in Chapter 3). This support could come in the form of institutional grants that can allow for faculty time to develop new courses, development of information technology to support education, support for student experiences in practice settings, and travel to meetings with others developing similar programs. Special attention should be paid to developing collaborations that can assure that the best of public health education is shared across schools, and re-invention of programs is kept to a minimum. A council parallel to the Council on Graduate Medical Education that is charged with continuous monitoring and improvement of the public health workforce development process could be an immense aid in this effort.

Development of Faculty

Federal agencies are in an ideal position to support faculty development. Creation of grants such as those already in place at NIH to support new biomedical and clinical researchers should be explored. Support might take the form of institutional grants (e.g., the NIH T32 model), given to an institution to develop or enhance research training in a specific area of study by funding predoctoral, postdoctoral, and short term research training. Other support could be through individual grants (e.g., the NIH K01 model), given to an experienced individual for 3–5 years of mentored research in a new area or using new research methods. Expanding the opportunities for early and mid-career faculty to do short-term rotations in government, private, or voluntary public health organizations would foster linkages between academic public health and practice, and the development of the research base. Fellowship programs to assist those who have extensive practice experience but lack the credentials for academic appointment could bring more practitioners into the ranks of those teaching public health.

Support for Students

At one time there were individual fellowship programs that provided financial support to persons employed in public health but lacking financial support to complete the M.P.H. degree. These programs have become scarce, making it more difficult for persons recruited to public health in mid-career, as is often the case, to obtain the additional training that would make them even more effective and that would encourage them to continue in public health practice. A new degree-oriented fellowship program might include support during pre-professional training to persons who make a commitment to specialty education and later practice, as well as support in collaboration with employing agencies for return-to-school programs for persons already working. Special attention should be paid to using this student support as a mechanism for increasing the racial and ethnic diversity of the public health workforce.

Continuing Education

While federal public health agencies have supported much technical and programmatic education for workers in federally funded public health program areas, the more recent work to make this education available via distance technology and to assure that it carries continuing education credits appropriate to the intended audience must be expanded. It may be that the CDC Public Health Training Network (described in Chapter 2) is best suited to acting as a mechanism for disseminating information about programs of suitable quality and connecting the workforce to the rich range of opportunities available. It is also critical that the federal agencies involved in public health practice attend to the continuing education of their own workforce, assuring that federal staff are not only technically competent in specific programs, but also that they are kept abreast of evolving organizational, ethical, and communication concerns of the practice community.

Technology Development

Much attention has been paid to the uneven availability of current information technology across the range of organizations engaged in the public health enterprise. CDC has paid particular attention to this and has invested significant funds in assuring at least a minimum of Internet connectivity for state and local public health agencies. As communications technology and teaching and learning technology continue to advance, federal agencies are in the best position to evaluate the applicability of these advances to the range of practice and educational settings and to provide incentives or other support for adoption of technologies deemed most likely to support an effective public health workforce. Such a role should not, however, be carried out in a vacuum but, instead, in partnership with practice agencies and schools.

Modeling

A final role that federal agencies can play in supporting the education of public health workers in the 21st century is modeling the best of what is known in recruitment, promotion, and retention policies. This would include assuring that all position descriptions for public health workers are based on public health competencies as developed by the field. Position announcements and recruitment should recognize (as many currently do) the importance of formal education in public health. When federal agencies hire persons who lack public health education for particular specialized tasks, on-the-job training, continuing education, and opportunities for formal education should include, at a minimum, a basic orientation to the core competencies in public health. Worker developmental activities should continue to include opportunities for short- and longer-term rotations to other practice agencies and to academic institutions, which are mechanisms through which the overall public health enterprise can be enriched and enlivened.

While the preceding discussion focused on HRSA and the CDC, the ideas are relevant to all branches of DHHS that are engaged in delivering one or more of the essential services of public health, and also to other federal agencies such as the Occupational Safety and Health Administration (OSHA) and the Environmental Protection Agency (EPA), and to the public health activities of the Department of Defense. The presence and leadership of these important federal partners in the public health enterprise cannot be overemphasized. Neither can the need for them to proceed in ongoing partnerships with the range of academic and practice agencies contributing to the same overall goal.

RECOMMENDATIONS

Local, state, and federal health agencies all play a critical role in educating public health professionals for the 21st century. Local health departments are the backbone of service in public health, meeting a broad range of public health needs of the diverse communities within their jurisdictions. To be able to engage in the most effective public health practice, practitioners in local health departments must be well educated and trained to fulfill their roles. To assure this is the case, we need to know what services they provide, and what skills and knowledge they need to ensure that their levels of competency are maintained and improved through appropriate training and educational opportunities.

At the state level, state health departments facilitate the implementation of the Essential Public Health Services either by carrying out these services directly or by supporting the efforts of the local public health agencies. One of these essential services is to assure a competent public health and personal care workforce. The state health department, in cooperation with local and federal public health agencies, has a major role to play in facilitating the competency of the public health workforce.

Finally, as described earlier, federal public health agencies are crucial to the education of public health professionals and the development of the public health workforce. Federal agencies can and must play important roles in many areas as discussed earlier in this chapter. These areas include public health research, development of academic programs, development of faculty, support for students, continuing education, technology development, and modeling. The importance of leadership and action at the federal level is critical to success in educating public health professionals if the public workforce is to meet the challenges of the 21st century.

Therefore, **the committee recommends that local, state, and federal health agencies:**

- **actively assess the public health workforce development needs in their state or region, including the needs of both those who work in official public health agencies and those who engage in public health activities in other organizations;**
- **develop plans, in partnership with schools of public health and accredited public health programs in their region, for assuring that public health education and training needs are addressed;**
- **develop incentives to encourage continuing education and degree program learning;**
- **engage in faculty and staff exchanges and collaborations with schools of public health and accredited public health education programs; and**
- **assure that those in public health leadership and management positions within federal, state, and local public health agencies are public health professionals with M.P.H. level education or experience in the ecological approach to public health.**

Assessment of workforce education and training needs and development and implementation of programs to meet these needs are major roles for local, state, and federal agencies. The issue of workforce training and competency is central to the success of any public health system. CDC and other public health agencies and organizations, including the National Association of County and City Health Officers (NACCHO), the Association of Schools of Public Health (ASPH), and the American Public Health Association (APHA), are examining the feasibility of creating a credentialing system for public health workers based on competencies linked to the Essential Public Health Services framework. Ideally, every state department of public health would be led by an individual who has formal credentials in public health.

While local, state, and federal agencies all play a role in developing a competent workforce, there is a role that is primarily the responsibility of federal agencies, that of providing funding to support efforts throughout the system. As detailed in Chapter 2, public health teaching, research, and infrastructure support were well funded during the 1960s and 1970s. Major reductions in funding occurred during the 1980s, with little or no improvement during the 1990s. Meanwhile tuition and other costs increased substantially, with the result that a reduction occurred in the amount of public health professional education actually provided.

Renewed interest in public health and the promise of increased funding may mean that needed investments to strengthen the public health infrastructure and workforce will be forthcoming. However we must ensure that funds are used for more than crash courses in a particular topic area (e.g., the current response to the threat of bioterrorism). We must also build the framework that will allow us, over the longer term, to ensure that public health professionals are prepared with the skills and knowledge necessary to improve population-level health. This means that increased funding must not only be a short-term response to a specific need but, instead, must be sustained over the long term. Such funding is crucial to developing the educational and research infrastructure necessary.

The committee has carefully considered the rationale and feasibility of implementing recommendations to significantly enhance federal funding for both public health education and leadership development and for public health research overall, including research on population health, public health systems, and public health policy. Investment in public health education is inadequate. Federal support for non-physician graduate-level public health training is minimal, as described in Chapter 2. Funding for residencies in preventive medicine is less than 1 percent of the overall federal investment in health professions training (about $1 million of the $300 million) (Glass, 2000). The report *Addressing the Nation's Changing Needs for Biomedical and Behavioral Scientists* (NRC, 2000) states that there is clear evidence of a decline in the number of M.D.s conducting research and concludes that enormous opportunities exist for more broadly trained investigators.

Therefore, **the committee recommends that federal agencies provide increased funding to**

- **develop competencies and curriculum in emerging areas of practice;**
- **fund degree-oriented public health fellowship programs;**
- **provide incentives for developing academic and practice partnerships;**

  • support increased participation of public health professionals in the education and training activities of schools and programs of public health; especially, but not solely, practitioners from local and state public health agencies; and

  • improve practice experiences for public health students through support for increased numbers and types of agencies and organizations that would serve as sites for practice rotations.*

It is extremely difficult to specify needed funding levels, given the weak data base on public health outcomes, public health programs, and public health education. The committee believes that federal funding for non-physician graduate public health education should receive a significant increase. The committee further believes that public health education for physicians should also increase significantly.

In terms of research funding, comparatively few resources have been devoted to supporting prevention research, community-based research, transdisciplinary research, or the translation of research findings into practice. Further, little public health systems research has been funded; such research is needed for better understanding of the factors that contribute to effective public health organization and service delivery. Current funding for research is focused almost entirely on two components of the ecological model of health—biologic determinants and medical cures. According to Scrimshaw and colleagues (2001), only 1–2 percent of the U.S. health care budget is spent on prevention and a like imbalance exists between funding for basic biomedical research and population-based prevention research. Actual causes-of-death analysis shows that at least 50 percent of mortality is due to factors other than biology and medical care (McGinnis and Foege, 1993). Because of this disproportionate spending away from preventive and public health interventions and research, we have lost major opportunities to prevent disease and disability, insofar as a substantial portion of mortality (estimated as high as 90 percent) and preventable disability is unrelated to health care per se (McGinnis and Foege, 1993).

CDC plays a major role in supporting public health research through both its intramural and its extramural research programs. *Intramural* (or CDC-directed) research is carried out within its laboratories or in the field in collaboration with local and state health departments. *Extramural* research, in which decision making regarding study approach rests with the grantee, consists of programs developed and administered independently through the CDC's Centers, Institutes, and Offices (CIOs). The

---

* Dr. Alan Guttmacher, because of his position as a federal employee, did not participate in discussions nor take a position regarding committee recommendations pertaining to federal funding.

CDC has three categories of extramural research programs: program or CIO-generated research, investigator-initiated research, and research centers of excellence. CDC is increasingly funding investigator-initiated research. Some components of CDC have been engaged in this activity for decades (e.g., National Institute for Occupational Safety and Health, which uses the NIH study section for peer review of its substantial extramural research program). The new CDC Director, with broad support from groups such as the Association of Schools of Public Health and the Association of Academic Health Centers, has identified expanded extramural investigator-initiated research among her highest priorities. This direction is fully consistent with CDC's prevention and population health mission. Despite the increase in funding for investigator-initiated research projects, this remains a relatively small endeavor.

The committee believes that significant steps to increase research funding are amply justified and warranted. Research!America, for example, with support from The Robert Wood Johnson Foundation, has launched a major effort to build support for health promotion and disease prevention research. The committee supports these efforts. However, given limited information on the full scope of the research agenda to be completed or the capacity of the public health enterprise to make rapid use of a sudden large increase, the following first efforts should be supported and their impact evaluated to identify the most fruitful area(s) for futher investment. Accordingly, **the committee recommends that**

- **there be a significant increase in public health research support (i.e., population health, primary prevention, community-based, and public health systems research), with emphasis on transdisciplinary efforts;**
- **the Agency for Healthcare Research and Quality spearhead a new effort in public health systems research;**
- **NIH launch a new series of faculty development awards ("K" awards) for population health and related areas; and**
- **there be a redirection of current CDC extramural research to increase peer reviewed investigator-initiated awards in population health, prevention, community-based, and public health policy research, reallocating a significant portion of current categorical public health research funding to competitive extramural grants in these areas.***

---

* Dr. Alan Guttmacher, because of his position as a federal employee, did not participate in discussions nor take a position regarding committee recommendations pertaining to federal funding.

Major change is called for in the funding of public health research. There must be increased emphasis on transdisciplinary research, public health prevention, systems, and policy research, and an assurance that traditional, single-discipline scientific review neither stalls nor thwarts the appropriate allocation of funds to scientifically meritorious transdisciplinary teams and proposals.

Local, state, and federal public health agencies form the backbone and the infrastructure for the public health system in the United States, and the workforce of these agencies is an essential component of that infrastructure. Public health professionals in these agencies, as well as in other organizations, must be appropriately educated to perform effectively. They must have the competencies necessary to serve as the front-line deliverers of public health services to diverse communities. They must be able to respond to rapidly changing needs, priorities, and technologies. They must have the knowledge and skills necessary to work effectively with many different disciplines, communities, and organizations. They must have an ecological perspective, grounded in the fundamental skills of public health.

Educating public health professionals to function effectively and to respond to the new and emerging challenges requires funding support. There is an old saying, "You get what you pay for." If we want high quality public health professionals, contributing through practice, teaching, and research to improved health in our communities, then we must be willing to provide quality support to the education of those professionals.

Conclusion

During the 20th century great achievements in public health contributed to reductions in both morbidity and mortality in the United States. Nonetheless, the primary foci of U.S. health efforts were on scientific advances and medical care tailored to the individual, and particularly to already manifest diseases. Accordingly, most investments in capacity building in the last century have paralleled the dominance of this biomedical model, with public (mostly federal) dollars directed at capital investments in hospitals and medical schools, and on research activities on these issues in academic medical centers (Boufford and Lee, 2001). Health investments in population-based or public health capacity building, whether in laboratories, information systems, research, or workforce development and training have lagged woefully behind (IOM, 1988).

A variety of forces—among them globalization, technologic and scientific advances, and rapid demographic shifts—are hastening the need to refocus attention and resources away from these traditional biomedical efforts toward those of population health. The committee has relied on an ecological model of health to shape the implications of these changes on public health workforce needs; developing a framework for education, training, and research based on the ecological model. The ecological model recognizes accumulating evidence that the health of individuals and the community is determined relatively little by health care per se and far more by multiple other factors, and by their interactions. These factors include biology (e.g., genetics), the social and physical environment, education, employment, and behavior (e.g., healthy behaviors such as exercise and unhealthy ones such as overeating).

We have developed a working definition of public health professionals. *A public health professional is a person educated in public health or a related
discipline who is employed to improve health through a population focus.* The
committee believes that well-educated public health professionals, who
have a real understanding of the multiple determinants of health and
their interactions (the ecological model), are critical to shaping new knowledge, programs, and policies relevant to both individual health and health
care, and to population health in the coming century. These professionals
must have a broad range of skills and information. They must be able to
understand and apply new advances in science (e.g., genetics), information, and computer science technology to public health practice and
learning (i.e., public health informatics). They must be proficient in communication in order to interact effectively with multiple audiences, to
understand and incorporate the needs and perspectives of culturally diverse communities in public health interventions and research, and to
inform policy. Further, public health professionals will need to apply new
approaches to research, approaches that involve practitioners, researchers, and the community in joint efforts to improve health and to understand global health issues that increasingly transcend national boundaries. Of course, public health professionals must be able to identify and
address the numerous ethical issues that arise in public health practice
and research.

Public health professionals come from a variety of professions and
are educated in a number of different types of institutions. Because education for all public health professionals, no matter where they are educated, must be both relevant to the challenges of the 21st century and of
high quality, the committee has focused its recommendations not just on
programs and schools of public health, but also on schools of medicine,
nursing, and other professional schools (e.g., law), as well as on local,
state, and federal public health agencies. Education, research, and practice linkages among these institutions must be fostered. Recent events,
particularly those of September 11, 2001, and their aftermath, have
brought public health and its professional practitioners from relative ob-
scurity to broad visibility. These events have dramatized the need to connect the spheres of health care and public health, both to each other and to
their interaction with the public. Clearly demonstrated was the need for
public health and health care sectors to be better able to characterize and
communicate risk and uncertainty.

The committee tackled the challenges faced by public health and its
professionals, given this moment in history, recognizing the opportunity
for public health to address many infrastructure and workforce needs
because of its increased visibility. As stated earlier in the report, previous
efforts to design truly effective systems of public health education generally foundered because of lack of political will, public disinterest, or pau-

city of funds. Despite the opportunities provided to public health in terms of resources and attention directed at disaster preparedness as a result of September 11, 2001, and the subsequent anthrax attacks, it is critical that this admittedly important issue not dwarf other challenges of public health and that necessary attention and support be given to strengthening the public health system, including educating public health professionals.

It is against this background that the committee developed its recommendations. Our recommendations are sometimes incremental, occasionally quite radical given our current baseline, but always grounded on a vision that if we lose sight of who will keep the public healthy, we will have lost an opportunity to improve the public's health during the 21st century.

References

AACN (American Association of Colleges of Nursing). 1999. A vision of baccalaureate and graduate nursing education: the next decade. *The Journal of Professional Nursing* 15(1): 59–65.

AIR (American Institutes for Research). 2002. *Teaching Cultural Competence in Health Care: A Review of Current Concepts, Policies, and Practices.* Washington, DC: Office of Minority Health, U.S. DHHS (U.S. Department of Health and Human Services).

Airhihenbuwa CO. 1995. *Health and Culture: Beyond the Western Paradigm.* Thousand Oaks, CA: Sage Publications.

Alcalay R, Ghee A, Scrimshaw S. 1993. Designing prenatal care messages for low-income Mexican women. *Public Health Reports* 108:354–262.

Altman DC. 1986. A framework for evaluating community-based heart disease prevention programs. *Social Science and Medicine* 22:479–487.

Anderson MB. 1999. Public health in medical education: where are we now? In: *Education for More Synergistic Practice of Medicine and Public Health.* New York: Josiah Macy, Jr., Foundation. Pp. 195–205.

ASPH (Association of Schools of Public Health)/Special Study Committee. 1966. *The Role of Schools of Public Health in Relation to Trends in Medical Care Programs in the United States and Canada.* Alan Mason Chesney Archives of the Johns Hopkins Medical Institutions.

ASPH. 1999. *Demonstrating Excellence in Academic Public Health Practice.* Washington, DC: ASPH.

ASPH. 2000. *1999 Annual Data Report: Applications, New Enrollments, and Students; Fall 1999 Graduates; 1998–1999 with Trends, 1989–1999.* Washington, DC: ASPH.

AUPHA (Association of University Programs in Health Administration). 2000. *Health Services Administration Education Directory of Programs 2001–2003.* Washington, DC: AUPHA.

Backstrom C, Robins, L. 1995. State AIDS policy making: perspectives of legislative health committee chairs. *AIDS & Public Policy Journal* 10(4):238–248.

Bandura A. 1986. *Social Foundations of Thought and Action: A Social Cognitive Theory.* Englewood Cliffs, NJ: Prentice Hall, Inc.

171

Barks-Ruggles E. 2001. The globalization of disease: when Congo sneezes, will California get old? *The Brookings Review*. [Online]. Available: http://www.brookings.edu/dybdocroot/press/REVIEW/fall2000/barks-ruggles.htm [accessed April 3, 2001].

Beaglehole R, Bonita R. 1998. Public health at the crossroads: which way forward? *Lancet*. Vol. 351:590–592.

Beauvais F, Trimble JE. 1992. The role of the researcher in evaluating American-Indian alcohol and other drug abuse. In: Orlandi MA, Weston R, Epstein LG, eds. *Cultural Competence for Evaluators: A Guide for Alcohol and Other Drug Abuse Prevention Practitioners Working With Ethnic/Racial Communities*. Rockville, MD: U.S. Department of Health and Human Services, Pp. 173–201.

Bell A. 1991. *The Language of News Media*. Cambridge, MA: Blackwell.

Berkman LF, Kawachi I. 2000. A historical framework for social epidemiology. In: Berkman LF, Kawachi I, eds. *Social Epidemiology*. Oxford, UK: Oxford University Press. Pp. 3–12.

Bialek R, Bialek J. 1999. Enabling the synergistic practice of public health and medicine through changes in public health education. In: *Education for More Synergistic Practice of Medicine and Public Health*. New York: Josiah Macy, Jr., Foundation. Pp. 220–237.

Bialek RG. 2001. *Council on Linkages Between Academia and Public Health Practice: Bridging the Gap Progress Report, July 1 through September 30*. Washington, DC: Public Health Foundation.

Blankenship KM. 2000. Structural interventions in public health. *AIDS* 14(Suppl 1):S11–21.

Blazer DG. 2000. Psychiatry and the Oldest Old. *American Journal Psychiatry* 157:1915–1924.

Blockstein AM. 1977. *Graduate School of Public Health, University of Pittsburgh, 1948–1974*. Pittsburgh: University of Pittsburgh.

Boden LI. 1996. Policy evaluation: better living through research. *American Journal of Industrial Medicine* 29(4):346–352.

Boufford JI, Lee PR. 2001. *Health Policies for the 21st Century: Challenges and Recommendations for the U.S. Department of Health and Human Services*. New York: Milbank Memorial Fund.

Braithwaite RL, Taylor SE. 1992. African-American health: an introduction. In: *Health Issues in the Black Community*. San Francisco: Jossey-Bass. Pp. 3–5.

Brandt AM, Gardner M. 2000. Antagonism and accommodation: interpreting the relationship between public health and medicine in the United States during the 20th Century. *American Journal of Public Health* May 90(5):707–715.

Brandt A, Kass AM. 1999. Collaboration and competition: tracing the historical relationship of medicine and public health in the 20th Century. In: *Education for More Synergistic Practice of Medicine and Public Health*. New York: Josiah Macy, Jr., Foundation. Pp. 23–35.

Brehm J. 1966. *A Theory of Psychological Reactance*. New York: Academic Press.

Brennan PF, Friede A. 2001. Public health and consumer uses of health information: education, research, policy, prevention, and quality assurance. In: Shortliffe EH, Perreault LE, eds. *Informations: Computer Applications in Health Care and Biomedicine, 2nd ed.* New York: Springer-Verlag. Pp. 397–420.

Brown P, Levinson SC. 1978. Universals in language use: politeness phenomena. In: Goody E, ed. *Questions and Politeness: Strategies in Social Interaction*. Cambridge, MA: Cambridge University Press. Pp. 56–289.

Brownson RC, Kreuter MW. 1997. Future trends affecting public health: challenges and opportunities. *Journal of Public Health Management Practice* 3(2):49–60.

Bullard RD, Johnson GS. 2000. Environmental justice: grassroots activism and its impact on public policy decision making. *Journal of Social Issues* 56(3):555–578.

Burris S. 1994. Thoughts on the law and the public's health. *Journal of Law, Medicine, and Ethics* 22(2):141–147.

Burris S. 1997. The invisibility of public health: population-level measures in a politics of market individualism. *American Journal of Public Health* 87(10):1607–1610.

Burris S, Gostin LO, Tress D. 2000. Public health surveillance of genetic information: ethical and legal responses to social risk. In: Khoury M, Burke W, Thomson E, eds. *Genetics and Public Health in the 21st Century: Using Genetic Information to Improve Health and Prevent Disease.* New York and Oxford: Oxford University Press. Pp. 527–548.

Burris S. 2002. Introduction: merging law, human rights and social epidemiology. *Journal of Law, Medicine, & Ethics* 30(4):498–509.

Burris S, Kawachi I, Sarat A. 2002. Integrating law and social epidemiology. *Journal of Law, Medicine, & Ethics* 30:510–521.

Butler RN. 1997. Population aging and health. *British Medical Journal* 315(7115):1082–1085.

Byrd ME. 1995. A concept analysis of home nursing. *Public Health Nursing* 12(2):83–89.

Callahan D, Jennings B. 2002. Ethics and public health: forging a strong relationship. *American Journal of Public Health* 92(2):169–176.

Carrese JA, Rhodes LA. 1995. Western bioethics on the Navajo reservation. *Journal of the American Medical Association* 274:826–829.

Carson, R. 1962. *Silent Spring.* Boston: Houghton Mifflin.

Casas JM. 1992. A culturally sensitive model for evaluating alcohol and other drug abuse prevention programs. In: Orlandi MA, Weston R, Epstein LG, eds. *Cultural Competence for Evaluators: A Guide for Alcohol and Other Drug Abuse Prevention Practitioners Working with Ethnic/Racial/Communities.* Rockville, MD: U.S. DHHS. Pp. 75–116.

CDC (Centers for Disease Control and Prevention). 1998. National Public Health Performance Standards. http://www.phppo.cdc.gov/nphpsp/index.asp.

CDC. 2001a. A global lifelong learning system: building a stronger frontline against health threats. In: *A Global and National Implementation Plan for Public Health Workforce Development.* Revision date: January 5, 2001.

CDC. 2001b. [Online]. Available: www.cdc.gov/PHTN/history.htm.

CDC. 2001c. [Online]. Available: www.phppo.cdc.gov/workforce.

CDC. 2001d. Genomics Workforce Competencies. [Online]. Available: www.cdc.gov/genomics/training/competencies/comps.htm.

Center for Health Policy. 2000. *The Public Health Workforce: Enumeration 2000.* New York: Columbia University School of Nursing.

Cirksena MK, Flora JA. 1995. Audience segmentation in worksite health promotion: a procedure using social marketing concepts. *Health Education Research* 10:211–224.

Clayton EW. 2000. Genetics, public health, and the law. In: Khoury MJ, Burke W, Thomson EJ, eds. *Genetics and Public Health in the 21st Century: Using Genetic Information to Improve Health and Prevent Disease.* New York: Oxford University Press. Pp. 489–503.

Cohen D, Spear S, Scribner R, Kissinger P, Mason K, Wildgen J. 2000. "Broken windows" and the risk of gonorrhea. *American Journal of Public Health* 90(2):230–236.

Collins FS. 1999. Shattuck lecture—Medical and societal consequences of the human genome project. *New England Journal of Medicine* July 1:341(1)28–37.

Collins FS, McKusick VA. 2001. Implications of the human genome project for medical science. *Journal of the American Medical Association* 285(5):540–543.

Committee on Professional Education. 1937. Public health degrees and certificates granted in 1936. *American Journal of Public Health* 27:1267–1272.

Community Health Resource Center. *Faculty-to-faculty Mentoring Program in Community Health.* [Online]. Available: http://www.nonpf.com/chmentor.htm [accessed July 30, 2000].

Conrad D. 2000. Bringing two worlds closer: a three-year review of council activities. *The Link* 14(1):1–4.

Cotton-Oldenburg NU. 2001. Impact of pharmacy-based syringe access on injection practices among injecting drug users in Minnesota, 1998 to 1999. *Journal of Acquired Immune Deficiency Syndromes,* 27(2):183–192.

Council on Linkages. 2001. *Core Competencies for Public Health Professionals.* Washington, DC: Public Health Foundation.

Covello VT. 1992. Risk communication: an emerging area of health communication research. In: Deetz SA, ed. *Communication Yearbook*. Vol. 15. Newbury Park, CA: Sage Publications. Pp. 359–373.

Dahlgren G, Whitehead M. 1991. Policies and strategies to promote social equity in health. Stockholm: Institute for the Futures Studies.

Danis M, Sepinwall A. 2002. Regulation of the Global Marketplace for the Sake of Health. *Journal of Law, Medicine, & Ethics* 30:667–676.

Davis MV, Dandoy S. 2001. *Survey of Graduate Programs in Public Health and Preventive Medicine and Community Health Education*. Final Report supported by ATPM/HRSA cooperative agreement 6U76AH000001. Washington, DC.

Day JC. 1996. Population projections of the United States by age, sex, race, and Hispanic origin: 1995 to 2050. In: U.S. Bureau of the Census. *Current Population Reports*. Washington, DC: U.S. Government Printing Office. Pp. 25–1130.

Duffy J. 1990. *The Sanitarians: A History of American Public Health*. Urbana, IL: University of Illinois Press.

Eisen K, Flake M, Wojciak A. 1994. How, where and when does theory meet practice? *The Link*. Baltimore, MD: Johns Hopkins University Health Program Alliance.

Elder JP, McGraw SA, Abrams DB, Ferreira A, Lasater TM, Longpre H, Peterson GS, Schwertfeger R, Carleton RA. 1986. Organizational and community approaches to community-wide prevention of heart disease: the first two years of the Pawtucket Heart Health Program. *Preventive Medicine* 15(2):107–117.

Emmons KM. 2000. Behavioral and social science contributions to the health of adults in the United States. In: *Promoting Health: Intervention Strategies from Social and Behavioral Research*. Washington, DC: National Academy Press.

Engs RC, Hanson DJ. 1989. Reactance theory: a test with collegiate drinking. *Psychological Reports* 64:1083–1086.

Epstein P. 1992. Cholera and the environment. *The Lancet* 339.

Erickson GP. 1987. Public health nursing initiatives: guideposts for future practice. *Public Health Nursing* 4(4):202–211.

Evans PP. 2002. (March 13). *An accreditation perspective on the future of professional public health preparation*. Presentation to the Institute of Medicine Committee on Educating Public Health Professionals for the 21st Century. Irvine, CA.

Evans RG, Stoddart GL. 1994. Producing health, consuming health care. In: Evans RG, Barer ML, Marmor TR, eds. *Why Are Some People Healthy and Others Not? The Determinants of Health of Populations*. New York: Aldine de Gruyter. Pp. 27–64.

Ewick P, Silbey S. 1998. *The Common Place of Law: Stories from Everyday Life*. Chicago: University of Chicago Press.

Farquhar JW, Fortmann SP, Maccoby N, Haskell WL, Williams PT, Flora JA, Taylor CB, Brown BW Jr., Solomon DS, Hulley SB. 1985. The Stanford five-city project: design and methods. *American Journal of Epidemiology* 122:323–334.

Fee E, Rosenkrantz B. 1991. Professional education for public health in the United States. In: Fee E, Acheson RM, eds. *A History of Education in Public Health: Health that Mocks the Doctors' Rules*. Oxford, UK: Oxford University Press. Pp. 230–271.

Fineberg HV, Green GM, Ware JH, Anderson BL. 1994. Changing public health training needs: professional education and the paradigm of public health. *Annual Review of Public Health* 15:237–257.

Fink L, Collins FS. 2000. The human genome project: evolving status and emerging opportunities for disease prevention. In: Khoury MJ, Burke W, Thomson EJ, eds. *Genetics and Public Health in the 21st Century: Using Genetic Information to Improve Health and Prevent Disease*. New York: Oxford University Press. Pp. 45–59.

Fischhoff B. 1999. Why (cancer) communication can be hard. *Journal of the National Cancer Institute Monographs* 25:7–13.

Fishbein M, Ajzen I. 1975. *Belief, Attitude, Intention, and Behavior.* Reading, MA: Addison-Wesley Publishing Company.

Flay BR. 1986. Efficacy and effectiveness trials (and other phases of research) in the development of health promotion programs. *Preventive Medicine* 15:451–474.

Freudenberg N, Golub, M. 1987. Health education, public policy and disease prevention: a case history of the New York City coalition to end lead poisoning. *Health Education Quarterly* 14(4):387–401.

Garrett L. 2000. *Betrayal of Trust: The Collapse of Global Public Health.* New York: Hyperion.

Gebbie KM. 1999. The public health workforce: key to public health infrastructure. *American Journal of Public Health* 89(5):660–661.

Gebbie KM, Hwang I. 2000. Preparing currently employed public health nurses for changes in the health system. *American Journal of Public Health* 90(5):716–721.

Gerzoff R, Brown C, Baker EL. 1999. Full-time employees of U.S. local health departments, 1992–1993. *Journal of Public Health Management and Practice* 5(3):1–9.

Ginzberg E, Dutka AB. 1989. *The Financing of Biomedical Research.* Baltimore: The Johns Hopkins Press.

Glasgow RE, Wagner EH, Kaplan RM, Vinicor F, Smith L, Norman J. 1999. If diabetes is a public health problem, why not treat it as one? a population-based approach to chronic illness. *Annals of Behavioral Medicine* 21:159–170.

Glass J. 2000. Physicians in the public health workforce. In: *Update on the Physician Workforce.* Council on Graduate Medical Education Resource Paper Compendium. Washington, DC: Health Resources and Services Administration, U.S. DHHS. Pp. 41–53.

Gold, SJ. 1992. Mental health and illness in Vietnamese refugees. *Western Journal of Medicine* 157:290–294.

Goodman RA, Lazzarini Z, Moulton AD, Burris S, Elster NR, Locke PA, Gostin LO. 2002. Other branches of science are necessary to form a lawyer: teaching public health law in law schools. *Journal of Law, Medicine, & Ethics* 30(2):298–301.

Goodman RM. 2000a. Bridging the gap in effective program implementation. *Journal of Community Psychology* 28(3):309–321.

Goodman RM. 2000b. Evaluation of community-based programs: an alternative perspective. In: Schneiderman N, Speers MA, Silva JM, Tomes H, Gentry JH. *Integrating Behavioral and Social Sciences with Public Health.* Washington, DC: American Psychological Association. Chapter 14.

Gordon LJ, McFarlane DR. 1996. Public health practitioner incubation plight: following the money trail. *Journal of Public Health and Policy* 17(1):59–70.

Gostin L, Lazzarini Z. 1997. *Human Rights and Public Health in the AIDS Pandemic.* New York and Oxford: Oxford University Press.

Gostin LO, Burris S, Lazzarini Z. 1999. The law and the public's health: a study of infectious disease law in the United States. *Columbia Law Review* 99(1):59–128.

Gostin LO. 2000. Public health law in a new century: part I: law as a tool to advance the community's health. *Journal of the American Medical Association* 283(21):2837–2841.

Gostin L. 2002. Public health law, ethics, and human rights: mapping the issues. In: Gostin L, ed. *Public Health Law and Ethics: A Reader.* Berkeley: University of California Press.

Grace CA. 1992. Cultural competence for evaluators: a guide for alcohol and other drug abuse prevention practitioners working with ethnic/racial communities. In: Orlandi MA, Weston R, Epstein, LG, eds. *Practical Considerations for Program Professionals and Evaluators Working With African-American Communities.* Rockville, MD: U.S. DHHS. Pp. 55–74.

Grayston JT. 1974. New approaches in schools of public health: the University of Washington School of Public Health and Community Medicine. In: Bowers JZ, Purcell EF, eds. *Schools of Public Health: Present and Future, A Report of a Macy Conference.* New York: Josiah Macy, Jr., Foundation. Pp. 49–59.

Green L, Daniel M, Novick L. 2001. Partnerships and coalitions for community-based research. *Public Health Reports 2001 Supplement 1* 116:20–30.

Green L, Kreuter M. 1999. *Health Promotion Planning: An Educational and Ecological Approach.* 3rd ed. Mountain View, CA: Mayfield Publishing.

Green LW, Mercer SL. 2001. Can public health researchers and agencies reconcile the push from funding bodies and the pull from communities? *American Journal of Public Health* 91(12):1926–1929.

Grzywacz JG, Fuqua J. 2000. The social ecology of health: leverage points and linkages. *Behavioral Medicine* 26(3):101–115.

Guarino MA. 1997. Business prospective: a complement to a successful public health agenda. *Journal of Public Health Management & Practice* 3(4):29–33.

Guttman N. 1997. Ethical dilemmas in health campaigns. *Health Communication* 9:155–190.

Hager M. 1999. *Education for More Synergistic Practice of Medicine and Public Health.* New York: Josiah Macy, Jr., Foundation.

Hall T. 1973. *Professional Health Manpower for Community Health Programs.* Chapel Hill, NC: School of Public Health of the University of North Carolina.

Halverson PK, Mays G, Kaluzny AD, House RM. 1997. Developing leaders in public health: the role of the executive training programs. *Journal of Health Administration Education* 15(2):87–100.

Hemenway D. 2001. The public health approach to motor vehicles, tobacco, and alcohol, with applications to firearms policy. *Journal of Public Health Policy* 22(4):381–402.

Hippocrates. 1939. (Circa 400 B.C.) Hippocrates on airs, waters, and places. In: *Great Books of the Western World.* Medical Classics. Pp. 111–119.

House JS, Williams D. 2000. Understanding and reducing socioeconomic and racial/ethnic disparities in health. In: Smedley BD, Syme SL, eds. *Promoting Health: Intervention Strategies from Social and Behavioral Research.* Washington, DC: National Academy Press. Pp. 81–124.

IOM (Institute of Medicine). 1988. *The Future of Public Health.* Washington, DC: National Academy Press.

IOM. 1997. *America's Vital Interest in Global Health.* Washington, DC: National Academy Press.

IOM. 1998. *From Generation to Generation: The Health and Well-Being of Children in Immigrant Families.* Washington, DC: National Academy Press.

IOM. 1999. *Gulf War Veterans: Measuring Health.* Washington, DC: National Academy Press.

IOM. 2000. *Promoting Health: Intervention Strategies from Social and Behavioral Research.* Washington, DC: National Academy Press.

IOM. 2001a. *Health and Behavior: The Interplay of Biological, Behavioral, and Societal Influences.* Washington, DC: National Academy Press.

IOM. 2001b. *New Horizons in Health.* Washington, DC: National Academy Press.

IOM. 2002. *Unequal Treatment: Confronting Racial and Ethnic Disparities in Health Care.* Washington, DC: National Academy Press.

Israel BA, Lichtenstein R, Lantz P, McGranaghan R, Allen A, Guzman JR, Softley D, Maciak B. 2001. The Detroit Community Academic Urban Research Center: development, implementation, and evaluation. *Journal of Public Health Management and Practice* 7(5):1–19.

Jacobs DR Jr, Luepker RV, Mittelmark MB, Folsom AR, Pirie PL, Mascioli SR, Hannan PJ, Pechacek TF, Bracht NF, Carlaw RW, et al. 1986. Community-wide prevention strategies: evaluation design of the Minnesota Heart Health Program. *Journal of Chronic Disease* 39:775–788.

James JS. 1998. GATT and the gap: how to save lives. *AIDS Treatment News* (307):1.

Jenkins J, Blitzer M, Boehm K, Feetham S, Gettig E, Johnson A, Lapham V, Patenaude A, Reynolds P, Guttmacher A. 2001. Recommendations of core competencies in genetics essential for all health professionals. *Genetics in Medicine* 3:155–159.

Kaferstein FK, Motarjemi R, Bettcher DW. 1997. Foodborne infectious disease control: a transnational challenge. *Bulletin of the World Health Organization* 3(4):503–510.

Kaplan GA, Everson SA, Lynch JW. 2000. The contribution of social and behavioral research to an understanding of the distribution of disease: a multilevel approach. In: Smedley BD, Syme SL, eds. *Promoting Health: Intervention Strategies from Social and Behavioral Research.* Washington, DC: National Academy Press. Pp. 37–80.

Kass NE. 2001. An ethics framework for public health. *American Journal of Public Health* 91(11):1776–1782.

Keitel MA, Kopala M, Adamson WS. 1996. Ethical issues in multicultural assessment. In: Suzuki LA, Meller PJ, Ponterotto JG, eds. *Handbook of Multicultural Assessment: Clinical, Psychological, and Educational Applications.* San Francisco: Jossey-Bass. Pp. 29–46.

Kennedy VC, Spears WD, Loe HD Jr., Moore FI. 1999. Public health workforce information: a state-level study. *Journal of Public Health Management Practice* 5(3):10–19.

Khoury MJ, the Genetics Working Group. 1999. From genes to public health: the applications of genetic technology in disease prevention. *American Journal of Public Health* 86(12):1717–1722.

Khoury MJ, Burke W, Thomson EJ, eds. 2000. *Genetics and Public Health in the 21st Century: Using Genetic Information to Improve Health and Prevent Disease.* New York: Oxford University Press.

Kickbusch I, Buse K. 2001. Global influences and global responses: international health at the turn of the 21st century. In: Merson MH, Black RE, Mills AJ, eds. *International Public Health: Diseases, Programs, Systems, and Policies.* Gaithersburg, MD: Aspen Publishers. Pp. 701–738.

Koplan JP, Fleming DW. 2000. Current and future public health challenges. *Journal of the American Medical Association* 284(13):1696–1698.

Krieger N. 2000. Discrimination and health. In: Berkman LF, Kawachi I, eds. *Social Epidemiology.* Oxford, UK: Oxford University Press. Pp. 36–75.

Lalonde M. 1974. *A New Perspective on the Health of Canadians.* Ottawa, ON: Ministry of Supply and Services.

Lasker RD, Humphreys Bl, Braithwaite WR. 1995. *Making a Powerful Connection: The Health of the Public and the National Information Infrastructure.* Washington, DC: Public Health Data Policy Coordinating Committee, U.S. Public Health Service.

Lasker RD. 1999. What to teach medical students about public health for synergistic practice. *Education for More Synergistic Practice of Medicine and Public Health.* Pp. 148–158.

Lasker R. 2001. Medicine and public health: the power of collaboration. In: Lee PR, Estes CL, eds. *The Nation's Health.* 6th ed. Sudbury, MA: Jones and Bartlett Publishers. Pp. 262–302.

Lee E. 1988. Cultural factors in working with Southeast Asian refugee adolescents. Special Issue: mental health research and service issues for minority youth. *Journal of Adolescence* 11:167–179.

Lee K. 1999. Globalization, communicable disease, and equity: a look back and forth. *Development* 42(4):35–39.

Lee K. 2000. The impact of globalization on public health: implications for the UK Faculty of Public Health Medicine. *Journal of Public Health Medicine* 22(3):253–262.

Levin BW. 2002. Public health and bioethics: the benefits of collaboration. *American Journal of Public Health* 92(2):165–167.

Liang AP, Renard PG, Robinson C, Richards TB. 1993. Survey of leadership skills needed for state and territorial health officers, United States, 1988. *Public Health Reports* 108(1): 116–120.

Link BG, Phelan J. 1995. Social conditions as fundamental causes of disease. *Journal of Health and Social Behavior* Spec No:80–94.

Maantay J. 2001. Zoning, equity, and public health. *American Journal of Public Health* 91(7): 1033–1041.

Macfarlane S, Racelis M, Multi-Muslime F. 2000. Public health in developing countries. *The Lancet* 356:841–846.

Maibach E, Parrott RL, Long DM, Salmon CT. 1994. Competencies for the health communication specialist of the 21st century. *American Behavioral Scientist* 38:351–360.

Mann JM. 1997. Medicine and public health, ethics and human rights. *Hastings Center Report* 27(3):6–13.

Marmot M. 2000. Multilevel approaches to understanding social determinants. In: Berkman L, Kawachi I, eds. *Social Epidemiology.* New York and Oxford, UK: Oxford University Press. Pp. 349–367.

Mattheos N, Schittek M, Attstrom A, Lyon HC. 2001. Distance learning in academic health education. *European Journal of Dental Education* 5:67–76.

Maurana C, Wolff M, Beck BJ, Simpson DE. 2000. Working with communities: moving from service to scholarship in the health professions. *Prepared for Discussion at Community-Campus Partnerships for Health's 4th Annual Conference.*

McCoullough DG. 1978. *The Path Between the Seas: The Creation of the Panama Canal, 1870–1974.* New York: Simon & Schuster.

McGinnis JM, Foege WH. 1993. Actual causes of death in the United States. *Journal of the American Medical Association* 170(18):2207–2211.

McLeroy KR, Bibeau D, Steckler A, Glanz K. 1988. An ecological perspective on health promotion programs. *Health Education Quarterly* 15(4):351–377.

McMichael AJ, Beaglehole R. 2000. The changing global context of public health. *The Lancet* 356:495–499.

McNeil JR. 2000. *Something New Under the Sun: An Environmental History of the Twentieth Century World.* New York: W.W. Norton. P. 339.

Mittelmark MB, Hunt MK, Heath GW, Schmid TL. 1993. Realistic outcomes: lessons from community-based research and demonstration programs for the prevention of cardiovascular diseases. *Journal of Public Health Policy* 14:437–462.

Mittelmark MB. 1999. The psychology of social influence and healthy public policy. *Preventive Medicine, 29*(6 Pt 2):S24–29.

MMF (Milbank Memorial Fund). 1976. *Higher Education for Public Health: A Report of the Milbank Memorial Fund Commission.* New York: Prodist.

Mo B. 1992. Modesty, sexuality, and breast cancer in Chinese American women. *The Western Journal of Medicine* 157:260–64.

Modeste NN. 1996. *Dictionary of Public Health Promotion and Education: Terms and Concepts.* Thousand Oaks, CA: Sage Publications.

Mullan F. 2000. Public health then and now. *American Journal of Public Health.* 90(5):702–706.

NACCHO (National Association of County and City Health Officials). 2001. *Local Public Health Agency Infrastructure: A Chartbook.* Washington, DC: NACCHO.

NASPAA (National Association of Schools of Public Affairs and Administration). 2002. [Online]. Available: http://www.naspaa.org/sur98_4.htm.

National Conference of State Legislatures. 2001. Updated November 2001 and January 2002. [Online]. Available: www.ncsl.gov.

Nestle M, Jacobson MF. 2000. Halting the obesity epidemic: a public health policy approach. *Public Health Report* Jan-Feb 115(1):12–24.

NIH (National Institutes of Health). 2002. [Online]. Available: www.niehs.nih.gov/translat/cbpr/cbpr.htm.

Novak WJ. 1996. *The People's Welfare: Law and Regulation in Nineteenth Century America.* Chapel Hill, NC: University of North Carolina Press.

NRC (National Research Council). 2000. *Addressing the Nation's Changing Needs for Biomedical and Behavioral Scientists.* Washington, DC: National Academy Press.

Nutbeam, D. 1996. Achieving "best practice" in health promotion: improving the fit between research and practice. *Health Education Research* 11(3):317–326.

Orlandi MS. 1992. The challenge of evaluating community-based prevention programs: a cross-cultural perspective. In: Orlandi MA, Weston R, Epstein LG, eds. *Cultural Competence for Evaluators: A Guide for Alcohol and Other Drug Abuse Prevention Practitioners Working with Ethnic/Racial/Communities.* Rockville, MD: U.S. DHHS. Pp. 1–22.

Padilla AM, Medina A. 1996. Cross-cultural sensitivity in assessment using tests in culturally appropriate ways. In: Suzuki LA, Meller PJ, Ponterotto JG, eds. *Handbook of Multicultural Assessment: Clinical, Psychological, and Educational Applications.* San Francisco: Jossey-Bass.

Pang, T. 2002. The impact of genomics on global health. *American Journal of Public Health.* 92(7):1077–1079.

Parmet WE, Robbins A. 2002. A rightful place for public health in American law. *Journal of Law, Medicine, & Ethics* 30(2):302–304.

Parrott R. 1995. Topic-centered and person-centered "sensitive subjects": recognizing and managing barriers to disclosure about health. In: Fuller LK, McPherson L, eds. *Communicating About Communicable Diseases.* Amherst, MA: HRD Press, Inc. Pp. 177–190.

Parrott R, Lewis D, Jones K, Steiner C, Goldenhar L. 1998a. Identifying feed and seed stores as a site to promote skin cancer control: a social marketing approach to agricultural health communications. *Journal of Agricultural Safety and Health* 98:149–158.

Parrott R, Monahan J, Ainsworth S, Steiner C. 1998b. Communicating to farmers about skin cancer: the behavior adaptation model. *Human Communication Research* 24:386–409.

Parrott R, Duncan V, Duggan A. 2001. Promoting patients' full and honest disclosure during conversations with health caregivers. In: Petronio S, ed. *Balancing the Secrets of Private Disclosures.* Mahwah, NJ: Lawrence Erlbaum Associates. Pp. 137–147.

Parrott R, Egbert N, Anderson J, Sefcovic E. 2002. Enlarging the role of environment in health campaigns. In: Dillard JP, Pfau M, eds. *Persuasion Handbook.* Thousand Oaks, CA: Sage. Pp. 633–660.

Paxman D, Lee P, Satcher D. 2000. Public health status at the beginning of the twenty-first century. In: Bruce T, Urangauru McKane S, eds. *Community-Based Public Health: A Partnership Approach.* Washington, DC: APHA (American Public Health Association).

PHLS (Public Health Leadership Society). 1999. *Development of the 21st Century Workforce: Leadership, Commitment, and Action—The Crucial Next Steps.*

Public Health Functions Steering Committee. 1994. *Public Health in America.* [Online]. Available: www.health.gov/phfunctions/public.htm.

QCPHNO (Quad Council of Public Health Nursing Organizations). [Online]. Available: http://www.phf.org/Link/quad_council.htm [accessed July 30, 2001].

QCPHNO. 1999. *Scope and Standards of Public Health Nursing Practice.* Washington, DC: American Nurses Association, American Nurses Publishing.

Rains JW, Barton-Kriese P. 2001. Developing political competence: a comparative study across disciplines. *Public Health Nursing* 18(4):219–224.

Reutter L, Williamson DL. 2000. Advocating healthy public policy: implications for baccalaureate nursing education. *Journal of Nursing Education* 39(1):21–26.

Richards TB, Croner CM, Rushton G, Brown CK, Fowler L. 1999. Geographic information systems and public health: mapping the future. *Public Health Reports* 114(4):359–360.

Richardson M, Casey S, Rosenblatt RA. 2001. Local health districts and the public health workforce: a case study of Wyoming and Idaho. *Journal of Public Health Management and Practice* 7(1):37–48.

Riegelman R, Persily NA. 2001. Health information systems and health communications: narrowband and broadband technologies as core public health competencies. *American Journal of Public Health* 91(8):1179–1183.

Rose G. 1985. Sick individuals and sick populations. *International Journal of Epidemiology* 14:32–38.

Rosenfeld LS, Gooch M, Levine OH. 1953. *Report on Schools of Public Health in the United States Based on a Survey of Schools of Public Health in 1950.* Public Health Service, U.S. DHEW Pub. No. 276. Washington, DC: U.S. Government Printing Office.

Rotz LD, Koo D, O'Carroll PW, Kellogg RB, Lillibridge SR. 2000. Bioterrorism preparedness: planning for the future. *Journal of Public Health Management Practice* 6:45–49.

Sarat A. 1990. ". . . the law is all over": power, resistance and the legal consciousness of the welfare poor. *Yale Journal of Law and the Humanities* 2:343–379.

Schmid TL, Pratt M, Howze E. 1995. Policy as intervention: environmental and policy approaches to the prevention of cardiovascular disease. *American Journal of Public Health* 85(9):1207–1211.

Schooler C, Chaffee SH, Flora JA, Roser C. 1998. Health campaign channels: tradeoffs among reach, specificity, and impact. *Human Communication Research* 24:410–432.

Schulz A, Parker E, Israel B, Fisher T. 2001. Social context, stressors, and disparities in women's health. *Journal of the American Medical Women's Association* 56:143–149.

Schulz AJ, Galea S, Krieger J. 2002. Special issue: community-based participatory research–addressing social determinants of health: lessons from the urban research centers. *Health Education & Behavior* 29(3).

Scott JD. 1990. *Domination and the Arts of Resistance: Hidden Transcripts.* New Haven, CT: Yale University Press.

Scrimshaw SC, White L, Koplan J. 2001. The meaning and value of prevention research. *Public Health Reports: 2001* Vol. 116 Supplement 1. 116:4–9.

Shepard WP. 1948. The professionalization of public health. *American Journal of Public Health* 38:145–153.

Sheps CG. 1976. *Higher Education for Public Health: A Report of the Milbank Memorial Fund Commission.* New York: Prodist.

Shine K. 1999. Perspectives of medicine. In: *Education for More Synergistic Practice of Medicine and Public Health.* New York: Josiah Macy, Jr., Foundation. Pp. 40–48.

Shinn M. 1996. Special issue: Ecological assessment. *American Journal of Community Psychology* 24(1).

St. Leger L. 2001. Schools, health literacy, and public health: possibilities and challenges. *Health Promotion International* 16(2):197–205.

Stokols D, Allen J, Bellingham RL. 1996. The social ecology of health promotion: implications for research and practice. *American Journal of Health Promotion* 10(4):247–251.

Strauss RP, Sengupta S, Quinn SC, Goeppinger J, Spaulding C, Kegeles SM, Millett G. 2001. The role of community advisory boards: involving communities in the informed consent process. *American Journal of Public Health* 91(12):1938–1943.

Strickland SP. 1972. *Politics, Science, and Dread Disease: A Short History of United States Medical Research Policy.* Cambridge, MA: Harvard University Press.

Sumartojo E. 2000. Structural factors in HIV prevention: Concepts, examples, and implications for research. *AIDS* 14(Suppl 1):S3–10.

Suzuki LA, Meller PJ, Ponterotto JG, eds. 1996. *Handbook of Multicultural Assessment: Clinical, Psychological, and Educational Applications.* San Francisco: Jossey-Bass.

Sweat MD. 1995. Reducing HIV incidence in developing countries with structural and environmental interventions. *AIDS* 9(Suppl A):S251–257.

Terris M. 1959. The changing face of public health. *American Journal of Public Health* 49:1119.

Thomas JC, Sage M, Dillenberg J, Guillory VJ. 2002. A code of ethics for public health. *American Journal of Public Health* 92(7):1057–109.

Tuckson RV. 1999. Perspectives on the current status of synergistic practice: some efforts, successes and failures. In: *Education for More Synergistic Practice of Medicine and Public Health.* New York: Josiah Macy, Jr., Foundation. Pp. 48–54.

Turnock BJ. 2001. *Public Health: What It Is and How It Works.* Gaithersburg, MD: Aspen Publishers, Inc.

Ullom-Muinich PD, Kallail KJ. 1993. Physicians' strategies for safeguarding confidentiality: the influence of community and practice characteristics. *Journal of Family Practice* 37: 445–448.

U.S. Census Bureau. 2001. *Overview of Race and Hispanic Origin, Census 2000 Brief.* Washington, DC: U.S. Bureau of the Census.

U.S. DHEW (U.S. Department of Health, Education, and Welfare). 1958. *Report of the National Conference on Public Health Training to the Surgeon General of the Public Health Service, July 28–30.* Washington, DC: DHEW.

U.S. DHHS (U.S. Department of Health and Human Services). 1988. *Bureau of Health Professions: Selected Summary Data on Fiscal Years 1980–1987 Awards.* Washington, DC: U.S. DHHS.

U.S. DHHS. 2000. *Healthy People 2010: Understanding and Improving Health.* Washington, DC: U.S. DHHS.

U.S. DHHS Agency for Healthcare Research and Quality. 2002a. *Addressing Racial and Ethnic Disparities in Health Care.* Fact Sheet. [Online]. Available: http://www.ahrq.gov/research/disparit.htm [accessed April 10, 2002].

U.S. DHHS Office of Minority Health. 2002b. *Teaching CulturalCompetencies in Health Care: A Review of Current Concepts, Policies, and Practices.* Washington, DC: U.S. DHHS.

Valente TW, Paredes P, Poppe PR. 1998. Matching the message to the process: the relative ordering of knowledge, attitudes, and practices in behavior change research. *Human Communication Research* 24:366–385.

Vega WA, VanOss-Marin B. 1997. Risk taking and abusive behavior. *Journal of Gender, Culture, and Health* 2:135–141.

Vega WA, Lopez SR. 2001. Priority issues in Latino mental health services research. *Mental Health Services Research* 3:189–200.

Wallack L, Dorfman L. 2001. Putting policy into health communication. In: Rice RE, Atkin CK, eds. *Public Communication Campaigns.* 3rd ed. Thousand Oaks, CA: Sage. Pp. 389–401.

Wedeking LA. 2001. The learning styles of public health nurses. *Capella University Ph.D. Dissertation.*

Weed DL, Mink PJ. 2002. Roles and responsibilities of epidemiologists. *Annals of Epidemiology* 12(2):67–72.

WHO (World Health Organization). 1948. *Constitution of World Health Organization Basic Documents.* Geneva: WHO

WHO. 2002. *Genomics and World Health: Report of the Advisory Committee on Health Research.* Geneva: WHO.

Williams KR, Scarlett MI, Jimenez R, Schwartz B, Stokes-Nielson P. 1991. Improving community support for HIV and AIDS prevention through national partnerships. *Public Health Reports* 106(6):672–677.

Winslow CEA. 1953. *The Accreditation of North American Schools of Public Health.* New York: American Public Health Association.

Woodward A, Kawachi I. 2000. Why reduce health inequalities? *Journal of Epidemiology and Community Health* 54(12):923–929.

Worthman CM. 1999. Epidemiology of human development. In: Panter-Brick C, Worthman CM, eds. *Hormones, Health, and Behavior: A Socio-ecological and Lifespan Perspective.* Cambridge: Cambridge University Press. Pp. 47–104.

Wortman C, Brehm J. 1975. Response to uncontrollable outcomes, an investigation of reactance theory and the learned helplessness model. In: Berkowitz L, ed. *Advances in Experimental Social Psychology.* New York: Academic Press. Pp. 278–336.

Yach D, Bettcher D. 1998. The globalization of public health, part I: threats and opportunities. *American Journal of Public Health* 88:735–738.

Yasnoff WA, O'Carroll PW, Koo D, Linkins RW, Kilbourne EM. 2000. Public health informatics: improving and transforming public health in the information age. *Journal of Public Health Management* 6(6):67–75.

Yasnoff WA, Overhage JM, Humphreys B, LaVenture M, Goodman K, Gatewood L, Reid J, Hammond E, Dwyer D, Huff S, Gotham I, Kukafka R, Loonsk J, Wagner M. 2001. A national agenda for public health informatics. *Journal of Public Health Management Practice* 7(6):1–21

Yen S. 1992. Cultural competence for evaluators working with Asian/Pacific Island-American communities: some common themes and important implications. In: Orlandi MA, Weston R, Epstein LG. eds. *Cultural Competence for Evaluators: A Guide for Alcohol and Other Drug Abuse Prevention Practitioners Working with Ethnic/Racial Communities*. Rockville, MD: U.S. DHHS. Pp.261–291.

Appendix A

School of Public Health
Catalogue Abstraction

SCHOOLS OF PUBLIC HEALTH CATALOG
ABSTRACTION SUMMARY

Twenty-nine (n = 29) school of public health catalogues were reviewed. Across these schools, 19 different graduate degrees are available, as shown in Table A-1. Table A-3 shows schools by master's degree offered; Table A-4 displays schools by doctoral degrees offered. Boxes A-1 through A-5 list the most frequently offered courses among accredited schools in five specialties: Epidemiology, Biostatistics, Environmental and Occupational Health, Community and Behavioral Health, and Health Services Policy and Administration.

At least one course in each of the five core areas (biostatistics, epidemiology, environmental health, health services administration, and social and behavioral sciences) is required for graduation in all the M.P.H. and Dr.P.H. programs. Most schools require or strongly recommend a field placement or practicum for both the professional and research degrees. The school of public health at the State University of New York at Albany

TABLE A-1   Graduate Degrees Available from Accredited Schools of Public Health

Master's Degree	Doctoral Degree
MPH, MA, MS, MASPH, MHA/MHS/MHSA, MOH, MHPE, MADH, MMM, MSEE, MSP, MCD	DrPH, PhD, ScD, DEnv, DPT, EdD

requires M.P.H. students to undertake two field placement internships while their Dr.P.H. students are required to rotate through four field placement internships.

More than half of the graduate programs require a comprehensive written or oral final examination for both the master and doctoral degrees. Fifteen schools require a comprehensive exam at the master level, an additional 4 schools offer a thesis or final exam option (Table A-2). Twenty-eight of the 29 schools require comprehensive exams at the doctoral level. (Note: Texas A&M does not offer any doctoral-level programs in public health.)

Most schools also require some sort of culminating capstone paper or project that incorporates all aspects of the degree training. For some schools, this final project is an extension of the field placement activity, where the student concludes the fieldwork, captures the experience in a paper, and presents the paper at the conclusion of the degree program.

TABLE A-2   Schools Requiring Comprehensive Exams at the Master Level

Required Comprehensive Exam	Berkeley	U. of Illinois-	St. Louis
	Boston U.	Chicago	UCLA
	Emory	Michigan	UNC
	Harvard	Minnesota	South Carolina
	Johns Hopkins	Oklahoma	South Florida
		Pittsburgh	
Thesis OR Exam Option	Ohio State		
	San Diego State		
	Tulane		
	UMass		

TABLE A-3   Schools by Master's Degree ($n = 29$)

Degree Awarded	School
MPH (29)	Berkeley, Boston U., Columbia, Emory, GW, Harvard, Johns Hopkins, U. of Illinois-Chicago, Iowa, Loma Linda, Michigan
MA (3)	Berkeley, Boston U., UMass
MS (24)	Berkeley, Boston U., Columbia, Emory, GW, Harvard, Johns Hopkins, U. of Illinois-Chicago, Iowa, Michigan, Minnesota
MSPH (6)	U. of Alabama-Birmingham, Emory, Loma Linda, Tulane, UNC, U. of South Florida
MHA/MHSA/MHS (14)	GW, Johns Hopkins, Iowa, Loma Linda, Michigan, Ohio State, Oklahoma, Pittsburgh, St. Louis U., Tulane, UNC
MOH (1) (Master of Occupational Health)	Harvard
MHPE (1) (Master of Health Promotion and Education)	Pittsburgh
MADH (1) (Master of Applied Development and Health)	Tulane
MMM (1) (Master of Medical Management)	Tulane
MSEE (1) (Master of Science in Environmental Engineering)	UNC
MSP/MCD (1) (Master of Speech Pathology/Master of Communication Disorders)	U. of South Carolina

TABLE A-4   Schools by Doctoral Degree ($n = 29$)

Degree Awarded	School
DrPH (17)	U. of Alabama-Birmingham, Berkeley, Columbia, GW, Harvard, Johns Hopkins, U. of Illinois-Chicago, Loma Linda, Michigan, Oklahoma, Pittsburgh, SUNY Albany, Tulane, UCLA, UNC, U. of South Carolina, UT-Houston
PhD (26)	U. of Alabama-Birmingham, Berkeley, Boston U., Columbia, Emory, GW, Harvard, Johns Hopkins, U. of Illinois-Chicago, Iowa, Michigan, Minnesota, Ohio State, Oklahoma, Pittsburgh, San Diego State, St. Louis U., Tulane, UCLA, UMass, UNC, U. of South Carolina, U. of South Florida, UT-Houston, Washington, Yale
ScD (4)	Boston U., Harvard, Johns Hopkins, Tulane
DEnv (1) Doctor of Environmental Science and Engineering	UCLA
DPT (1) Doctor of Physical Therapy	U. of South Carolina
EdD (1)	U. of South Carolina

BOX A-1   Most Offered Courses Among Accredited Schools in Epidemiology

Principles of Screening
Principles of PH Surveillance
Principles of Epi
Observational Epi
Epi Methods
Epi Theory
Logic, Causation, and Probability
Statistics for Epidemiology
Survey Design and Analysis
Techniques of Survey Research
Data Collection
Design and Conduct of Clinical Trials
Design and Management of Epi Studies
Design and Analysis of Epi Studies
Meta-Analysis
Epi Analysis of Outbreaks
Genetics in Epi
Problems of Design in Epi Studies
Problems of Measurement in Epi
Epi Modeling
Grantwriting for PH

Epi Topics
  Ca Epi
  EOH Epi
  CVD Epi
  Infectious Disease Epi
  Chronic Disease Epi
  Hospital Infections
  Reproductive Epi
  HIV/AIDS Epi
  Violence Epi
  Aging Epi
  Pediatric Epi
  Epi of STDs
  Psychiatric Epi
  Parasitic Disease Epi
  Trauma Epi

BOX A-2 Most Offered Courses Among Accredited Schools in Biostatistcs

Biometry
Biostatistic Methods
Data Analysis
Research Methods
Probability Theory
Statistical Methods for Sample Surveys
Survival Analysis
Stochastic Processes
Statistical Inference
Causal Inference
Regression Techniques and Analysis
Logistical Regression
Linear Regression Models

Regression and Analysis of Variance
Time Series Analysis
Statistical Analysis of Categorical Data
Longitudinal Data Analysis
Bayesian Inference and Analysis
Multivariate Statistics
Nonparametric Statistics
Principles of Applied Sampling Methods
Demographic Methods
Biostatistic Computer Applications
    (SAS/S-Plus)
Principles of PH Informatics
Database Management Systems
Health Info Systems

BOX A-3 Most Offered Courses Among Accredited Schools in Environmental and Occupational Health

Principles, Practices, and Policy
Prin of Occupational/
    Environmental Disease
Environmental Health Policy
Occupational Health Policy
Principles of Risk Assessment
Exposure Assessment and Control
Management of Natural Resources
Applications of Environmental
    Management
PH Issues in Disasters
PH Implications of War and Terrorism

Air Quality
Principles of Industrial Ventilation
Ventilation and Indoor Air Quality
Respiratory Physiology
Air Pollution

Toxicology
Toxicology
Toxicokinetics
Toxicodynamics
Molecular Toxicology
Genetic and Systemic Toxicology
Transport and Fate of Environmental Agents
Environmental Sampling and Analysis

The Physical Environment
Control of Exposure to Physical and
    Chemical Hazards
Management of Hazardous Materials
Occupational Safety and Ergonomics
Noise and Other Physical Agents
Industrial Hygiene
Industrial Safety and Injury Prevention
Injury Control and Prevention

Water Quality
Water Environment
Water Quality Management
Water and Wastewater Treatment
Water Pollution and Health
Waterborne Diseases
Applied Ecology

BOX A-4   Most Offered Courses Among Accredited Schools in Community and Behavioral Health

Foundations
Foundations of Community Health
  Sciences
Principles of PH Practice
Program Planning, Development,
  and Evaluation
Community Health Needs Assessment
Measuring Population Health

Health and Society
Society and Health
Social and Cultural Perspectives in PH
Inequality and Health
Race, Ethnicity, and Health
Health Problems of Minority
  Populations

Maternal and Child Health
Foundations of MCH
PH Practice in MCH
Programs in MCH
MCH Policymaking
Family Planning Policies and Programs
Perinatal Health
Children's Health
Adolescent Health
Social Services for Children and
  Families
Child Abuse and Neglect
Women's Health
Sexuality, Gender, and Health
MCH in Developing Countries

The Aging Population
Aging and PH
Geriatrics and Gerontology
Social Aspects of Aging
Chronic Illness and Aging
Health Policy and the Aged
Dying, Grief, and Hospice

Nutrition Sciences
Food Science
Food Sanitation and Safety
Nutrition Assessment
Nutrition in the Life Cycles
Nutrition Policies and Programs
Food and Nutrition Planning
Nutrition and Chronic Disease

Communications
Health and Risk Communication
Mass Communication in PH
Health Communication Campaigns
Health Marketing

Ethical Considerations
PH Ethics
Population Ethics
Research Ethics and Integrity
Health and Human Rights
PH in Complex Humanitarian
  Emergencies
Disaster Management

Health Education
Health and Behavior
Health Behavior Theory
Behavioral Factors in Disease
  Prevention
Community Health Education
School Health
Health Education Program
  Administration
Administration of Health Programs
Social Marketing in Health Education
Patient Education in the Health Care
  Delivery System
Preventive Health
Worksite Health Promotion
Health Promotion and Disease
  Prevention

International Health
Fundamentals of International Health
International Policy
Social and Behavioral Aspects of IH
Health Svcs Research in Developing
  Countries
Health in Developing Areas
Nutrition in the Third World

Behavioral Health
Drugs and Society
Substance Abuse Education and
  Prevention
Substance Abuse Policy Perspectives
Violence as a PH Problem
Mental Illness as a PH Problem

BOX A-5 Most Offered Courses Among Accredited Schools in Health Services Policy and Administration

Health Policy
Role of Government in Health Policy
Health Care Politics and Policy
Health Planning and Policy
Political Economy of Health Care
The Economics of Health Policy
Health Policy Analysis
Health Policy and Resource Allocation
Health Policy and Aging

Health Care Organization
Health Care Systems
Health Regulation and Planning
The US Health Care System
Theories of Organization and
   Management
Organization of Health Care Services
Rural Health and Health Services
Management of Health Care
   Organizations
Hospital Management and Administration
Ambulatory Care
Managed Care
Long-term Care Management and
   Administration
HMOs and Managed Care
EMS and Trauma Systems

Health Law
Fundamentals of PH Law
The Role of Law in PH Policy
Legal Aspects of Health Admin
Legal Problems in Health Facility
   Administration
Ethics in PH Research and Policy
Government Regulations in Health Care

Health Economics and Finance
Payment Systems of Health Care
   Organizations
Health Care Economics
Health Care Finance
Cost-Effectiveness and Cost-Benefit
   Analysis in PH
Health Care Budgeting and Strategic
   Planning
Financial Management in
   Health Care Orgs
Impact of Insurance on Health Care
Health Insurance Principles and
   Programs
Competition, Regulation, and
   Insurance

Health Care Delivery
Marketing of Health Services
Human Resource Management in
   Health Svcs
Medical Care Organization and
   Delivery
Delivery of Health Care Services
Delivery of Mental Health Services
Practical Problems in Health Svcs
   Admin
Leadership in PH Practice

Quality of Health Care
Health Svcs Research
Understanding Health Care Quality
Quality of Care
Quality Management in Health Care
Quality Measurement in HC
Quality Improvement in HC

Appendix B

School of Public Health
Survey Instrument

Dear Dean,

The IOM Committee on Educating Public Health Professionals for the 21st Century has been asked by the Robert Wood Johnson Foundation to assess the past and current state of public health professional education and training and contrast it to future practice needs. The committee's findings will be used to develop a framework for how, over the next five to ten years, education, training, and research in the schools of public health can be strengthened to meet the needs of future public health professionals to improve population health.

As part of its deliberations, the committee has been asked to answer the question, "What progress have schools of public health made in responding to the recommendations of the 1988 IOM report, *The Future of Public Health*?" The attached survey has been developed with that question in mind since the committee believes that those in the best position to answer the question are the schools of public health.

Each recommendation as stated in the 1988 IOM report is followed by one or more questions. A comment space at the end of the questionnaire is provided for additional information you may wish to share with the committee. We have avoided asking questions about information that is available elsewhere, such as through CEPH.

We appreciate your time and willingness to complete this survey. The information you provide will assist the IOM committee to better understand the current status of public health education and the progress made in preparing graduates of these programs. **Please return your responses by March 18, 2002 to:**

> Marc Ehman (FO 3021)
> Research Assistant
> Institute of Medicine
> 2001 Wisconsin Ave, NW
> Washington, DC 20007
> Email: Mehman@nas.edu

If you have any questions about this questionnaire, please contact

> Lyla M. Hernandez
> IOM Study Director
> Email: Lhernand@nas.edu
> Telephone: 518-478-2216

Sincerely yours,

Kristine Gebbie,   Linda Rosenstock
Co-Chair   Co-Chair

Name of School _____

Please list the number of faculty at your school in each of the following categories

1. Full-time faculty with primary appointment in the school of public health _____

2. Full-time faculty with primary appointment in another school _____

Recommendation 1: "Schools of public health should establish firm practice links with state and/or local public health agencies so that significantly more faculty members may undertake professional responsibilities in these agencies, conduct research there, and train students in such practice situations. Recruitment of faculty and admission of students should give appropriate weight to prior public health experience as well as to academic qualifications."

1. Do faculty from the school undertake professional responsibilities in a state health department?
    YES _____   NO _____

- If yes, please check the kinds of work undertaken. Check only those that have occurred within the past 5 years.

Requested research projects	☐
Technical assistance	☐
Ongoing professional responsibilities (e.g., serve as local epidemiologist or health officer)	☐
Staff development or training	☐
Appointment to professional advisory committee	☐
Other:_____	☐

- During the past 12 months what would you estimate to be the percent of your faculty engaged in such activity?

2. Is there an opportunity for students to earn credit hours for practice in a state health department?   YES _____ NO _____

- Is there a requirement that students undertake a period of work in a state health department?   YES _____ NO _____

- What do you see as barriers to student practice in state health departments?

- During the past 12 months, what would YOU estimate to be the percentage of your students who have undertaken a period of work in state health departments?

3. Do faculty from the school undertake professional responsibilities in a local health department?
   YES _____ NO_____ N.A. _____ (no local health dept.)

- If yes, please check the kinds of work undertaken. Check only those that have occurred within the past 5 years.

Requested research projects	☐
Technical assistance	☐

Ongoing professional responsibilities
(e.g., serve as local epidemiologist or
health officer) ☐
Staff development or training ☐
Appointment to professional
advisory committee ☐
Other:_____ ☐

- During the past 12 months what would you estimate to be the percent of your faculty engaged in such activity?

4. Is there an opportunity for students to earn credit hours for practice in a local health department?
   YES _____ NO _____ N.A. _____ (no local health dept.)

- Is there a requirement that students undertake a period of work in a local health department?
   YES _____ NO _____ N.A. _____ (no local health dept.)

- What do you see as barriers to student practice in local health departments?

- During the past 12 months, what would you estimate to be the percentage of your students who have undertaken a period of work in local health departments?

5. How important is professional experience in weighing student applications for admission to the school?

   Very important _____
   Important _____
   Somewhat important _____
   Not important _____

6. How important is practice-based activity (i.e., non-research, non-academic) experience in recruiting faculty for the school?

   Very important_____
   Important_____
   Somewhat important_____
   Not important _____

Recommendation 2: "Schools of public health should fulfill their potential role as significant resources to government at all levels in the development of public policy."

1. In your estimate, in which of the activities below has the school been engaged during the past 5 years? Please check all that apply.
   Policy development for legislative body ____
   Public health advocacy with state government ____
   Public health advocacy with local government ____
   Research requested by state policy makers ____
   Research requested by local policy makers ____
   Public health workforce development ____
   Other:_____

2. What do you see as barriers to your school being able to achieve its potential in this area?

Recommendation 3: "Research in schools of public health should range from basic research in fields related to public health, through applied research and development, to program evaluation and implementation research."

What, in your estimation, is the percent of research conducted in your school that you would characterize as:

___ Basic or fundamental research: research conducted for the purpose of advancing our knowledge.
___ Applied research: research designed to use the results of other research (e.g., basic research) to solve real world problems.
___ Translational research: research on approaches for translating results of other types of research to community use.
___ Evaluative research: the use of scientific methods to assess the effectiveness of a program or initiative.

Recommendation 4: "Schools of public health should take maximum advantage of training resources in their universities, for example, faculty and courses in schools of business administration, and departments of physical, biological, and social sciences."

Please circle below the other departments/schools where students of your school of public health may take courses that count toward their public health degree.

Medicine	YES	NO
Nursing	YES	NO

Dentistry	YES	NO
Pharmacy	YES	NO
Health sciences	YES	NO
Law	YES	NO
Social work	YES	NO
Academic health centers	YES	NO

Other, please specify _____

What is your estimate of the frequency with which such activities have been undertaken during the past 5 years?

Often _____

Sometimes _____

Not very often _____

Please list barriers to such activity

Recommendation 5: "Schools of public health should extend their expertise to advise and assist with the health content of educational programs of other schools and departments of the university."

Please circle below the other departments/schools where faculty of your school of public health have assisted in development of educational programs.

Medicine	YES	NO
Nursing	YES	NO
Dentistry	YES	NO
Pharmacy	YES	NO
Health sciences	YES	NO
Law	YES	NO
Social work	YES	NO
Academic health centers	YES	NO

Other, please specify _____

What is your estimate of the frequency with which such activities have been undertaken during the past 5 years?

Often _____

Sometimes _____

Not very often _____

Please list barriers to such activity

Recommendation 6: "Schools of public health should encourage and assist other institutions (e.g., colleges, universities, health departments) to prepare appropriate, qualified public health personnel for positions in the field. When educational institutions other than schools of public health undertake to train personnel for work in the field, careful attention to the scope and capacity of the educational program is essential."

Please circle below the other departments/schools where faculty of your school of public health have assisted in development of educational programs.

Medicine	YES	NO
Nursing	YES	NO
Dentistry	YES	NO
Pharmacy	YES	NO
Health sciences	YES	NO
Law	YES	NO
Social work	YES	NO
Academic health centers	YES	NO

What is your estimate of the frequency with which such activities have been undertaken during the past 5 years?

Often _____

Sometimes _____

Not very often _____

Please list barriers to such activity

Recommendation 7: Schools of public health should strengthen their response to the needs for qualified personnel for important, but often neglected, aspects of public health such as the health of minority groups and international health."

Does your school offer courses largely devoted to the following areas? Please check all that apply and attach course(s) outline or description.

Cultural competencies _____

Ethics _____

Health disparities _____

Social justice _____

Human rights _____

International or global health _____

Social epidemiology _____

Recommendation 8: "Education programs for public health professionals should be informed by comprehensive and current data on public health personnel and their employment opportunities and needs."

1. Does your school conduct an alumni survey?
    YES _____ NO _____

    If you are willing to share the results of that survey, please enclose a copy of the analysis.

2. Does your school conduct exit surveys?
    YES _____ NO _____

    If you are willing to share results of these surveys, please enclose a copy of the results of your most recent survey.

3. Please list other approaches you have used to collect data on public health personnel and their employment opportunities and needs. Please include copies of these reports, to the extent that you wish to share that information.

Finally, the committee would like to ask you to let us know what you believe to be the most important challenges and opportunities facing schools of public health and M.P.H. programs over the next 10 years. (Attach additional page if needed.)

We very much appreciate your willingness to participate in this survey and we will be happy to share the results of the analysis of responses as soon as it is available. Thank you.

Appendix C

Organizational Input

ASPH Answers for the IOM Study on Educating Public Health Professionals for the 21st Century

1.   Why would your organization or the members of your organization consider hiring someone with a public health education?

(a) The <u>Association of Schools of Public Health</u> (ASPH) has a mission to: strengthen, coordinate, and promote the education, research, and service activities of the 31 accredited schools of public health. In 2000, the then 28 member schools launched almost 6,000 masters and doctoral graduates into the workforce. Current association policy calls for graduates from an ASPH member school to fill key staff management positions. This policy ensures that the ASPH staff leadership are familiar with schools of public health and are well-versed in the core areas of public health; and,

(b) <u>Graduate schools of public health</u> are exceptionally interdisciplinary institutions that hire and promote faculty and staff who represent fields ranging from anthropology to zoology. Core doctoral training in public health, however, is required for most faculty positions. Individuals who have been academically prepared in other fields, nonetheless, often have a masters-level degree in public health.

2.   What is the minimum knowledge you or your organization's members expect from someone with a public health education?

ASPH and its members consider the master of public health (M.P.H.) degree the basic professional public health degree. The M.P.H. is the most commonly awarded degree at schools of public health (accounting for 63 percent of degrees awarded in 1999–2000). Other masters-level degrees that are conferred in schools of public health (e.g., M.S., M.H.A./M.H.S.A., and M.S.P.H.) are valued as comparable professional degrees to the M.P.H.

While graduates of schools of public health practice in every imaginable industry and setting in a field that becomes increasingly more complex and inter- and multi-disciplinary every year, there remain five core areas of knowledge that schools of public health must make available to masters and doctoral students: biostatistics, epidemiology, environmental health sciences, health services administration, and social and behavioral sciences. Individual schools may make other coursework mandatory, at their discretion. For example, the Biological Basis for Public

Health, Community Health Sciences, and Health Law are three required courses at different ASPH member schools.

More and more, schools of public health are tailoring flexible programs to assure that curricula continually evolve to meet new and emerging needs in research and practice. For example, residential and distance learning opportunities are commonly found at both degree and non-degree levels, including: management science, leadership for community health improvement, and emergency preparedness.

3.   What do you or your organization's members view as the most important areas for education for public health professionals?

The challenge for schools of public health (SPH) is that our graduates are employed in an increasingly broad variety of settings and venues. There is no longer such a thing as a "classic" student in an SPH, as in years past when the average student was a clinician in professional practice who sought an M.P.H. in order to work in a health department or similar setting. We know that very few students today go to work in state and local health agencies and, in the absence of accurate data that would track where our graduates go to work, SPH need to train emerging health professionals to practice in every imaginable worksite. Moreover, the standard academic research focus, once the sole clear-cut purpose of SPH located in research universities, while still the bedrock of academic public health, is making room for investigative approaches that incorporate perspectives from other disciplines and pedagogies, as well as from communities themselves.

Over the last two and a half years, the ASPH Education Committee has been discussing and refining a draft conceptual framework of the key perspectives, skills, and settings in which M.P.H. students should become competent upon graduation from an ASPH member school. The original framework that is currently under discussion, while not discarding the five core knowledge areas mentioned above, presents a crosscutting schema for graduate public health education. This process is still underway and is anticipated to result in a consensus around the core *areas* of competence during the spring of 2002.

4.   What do you or your organization's members see as the strengths and challenges facing public health education today?

The ASPH Strategic Planning Committee recently identified the key strategic considerations that define the current external and internal environments for the association. This process produced a list of organizational strengths and weaknesses and a list of environmental opportunities and threats as they relate to ASPH. Excerpted below are the points relative to graduate public health education:

Strengths

- There is a large pool of talented faculty at schools of public health who can lead the education of emerging public health professionals as well as the training of public health practitioners
- Federal agencies have recognized schools of public health as educational institutions that provide valuable research and teaching
- M.P.H. is a shared, well-recognized "product"
- The 31 schools of public health represent a vast resource for public health education, representing an array of institutions with a diverse portfolio of degrees and activities
- The trend towards competency-based education and performance standards
- Changes in the healthcare industry, such as the trend towards managed care and the increasing focus on population health

Weaknesses

- Cost of graduate public health education, plus low starting remuneration for many fields
- Tensions exist between academic and practice activities
- Signature doctoral degree (Dr.P.H.) has low status and no clear definition

Environmental opportunities

- Increased prominence of public health following the World Trade Center disaster and the use of anthrax as a bioterrorist weapon
- Recognition of the need to support public health infrastructure
- Growing government and foundation support for health-related research
- Federal commitment to reducing health disparities
- Increasing public emphasis on disease prevention and health promotion
- Application of public health methods to key issues in medical care
- Development of coalitions to advocate for major increases in funding
- Training and credentialing of the public health workforce
- Application of new technologies, including the World Wide Web, which has broadened access to graduate public health education and increased research possibilities

- Potential for new partnership with medical and other schools
- Expanding job market for SPH graduates
- Globalization
- Marketing potential of accreditation
- Response to growth of the aging population

Environmental threats

- Weak public understanding of, and support for, "public health"
- No respect for value of academic public health
- Lack of faculty diversity, which may hinder the recruitment and retention of underrepresented minority faculty and students
- Adverse government policies and funding priorities
- Reductions in federal funding for public health education and practice
- The difficulty in staying current with the increasingly rapid pace of change

5. What, in your opinion, are changes that might occur in the next 10 years that will call for new skills/knowledge to be added to public health professional training?

As far as graduate public health education is concerned, a number of changes are influencing the way that the 31 accredited schools of public health educate graduates:

(a) Diversity of Practice Setting

Each year brings new opportunities for public health practice and concomitant new titles and scopes of work for graduates of schools of public health. The diversity of duties for which public health professionals have primary or partial responsibility has yet to be accurately enumerated. As SPH gain more understanding of where our graduates practice, analyze job trajectories, and consider implications for graduate public health education as well as needs for lifelong learning, we will continue to refine the way we prepare students for successful practice in the "real world."

(b) Demographic Changes in Student Bodies

The classic student in a school of public health used to be a white, clinically trained doctor or nurse who pursued a M.P.H. in order to practice at the level of a health department or other similar setting. Students of public health today are increasingly younger, with less work experience, and more varied in the academic disciplines and the perspectives they bring to the profession. Students who seek current training in public health are also more diverse regarding ethnicity, race, age, and culture. While men used to outnumber women in SPH, today women represent over two-thirds of matriculates. Many students seek a part-time or other flexible educational experience. The challenge in this area results from maintaining a balance in trying to attract students into SPHs who have some prior public health experience while succeeding in tapping into the talents of younger, inexperienced students and shaping them into effective public health professionals.

(c) More Interdisciplinary and Interpersonal Context for Public Health Work

Public health professionals joining the work force today interact even more closely than those in years past with health sciences professionals and others whose primary goals may seem distal to public health. Colleagues in fields as varied as the transportation or building industries, or the prison or welfare systems, increasingly focus on (or can be encouraged to consider) the health and safety of their constituencies and the general public. Professionals in these fields may be experiencing changes in their areas of work as rapid and pervasive as in the core public health areas. Honing interpersonal skills and employing team approaches to decision making and problem solving have taken on a whole new meaning for public health professionals. Public health professionals must now also work in partnership with communities of all types (including mobilizing the "communities" of business, government, science, media, etc.) as well as serve communities that experience the greatest burden of disease. They must focus their efforts on community-wide results, and do so without constituencies of grateful individual patients to laud and support their work. They must account for the powerful influence within communities of cultural and normative values.

Further, public health practice has expanded to include virtually every sector of society, from agriculture to zoology, and it pervades people's lives in ways that few individuals thoroughly appreciate. Public health work is ubiquitous, and one may encounter large numbers of professionals with graduate public health training in community-based organizations, not-for-profit agencies, business, the insurance industry, foundations, high-tech operations, and every imaginable venue for providing conventional and alternative prevention services.

In response to this reality, applied learning opportunities, such as internships, fellowships, and interdisciplinary team projects, have become more available in schools of public health.

(d) Changing Fundamentals of Practice

The concepts, principles, and methods underlying the work of public health have evolved dramatically in recent decades, and this rapid development shows no sign of stopping. Interest in the social and behavioral sciences and epidemiology, in particular, is expanding as a result of research advances and improvements in methodologies, including the genomic, molecular, and biological sciences. This acceleration in basic scientific discoveries also speeds up the need for their continuous translation through public health disciplines into safe, practical, accessible benefits for all. The legal, ethical, and social issues attending new findings are profound. Deciding how to harness new knowledge in ways that protect, preserve, and promote what is strong and productive in social, cultural, and moral terms requires full public participation and discourse. Ensuring community involvement in decision-making—the hallmark of the public health process—is becoming an even more important, sensitive, and complex endeavor. Cultural competency has been identified as a critical skill for all public health practitioners, particularly as the United States evolves towards a more diverse society.

The worldwide impact of new communication technologies and computer-based tools transforming information exchange in all its aspects brings great promise for improving the health of the public. With these technologies, however, has come the limitless potential for disseminating misinformation and an unfortunate capacity to extol the popular rather than the accurate, especially as it relates to heath. Attending the exponential growth in the availability of information is the need for people to sort it out, to be more analytical in their use of it, and apply it more effectively in problem solving. Using information that is related to clinical treatment and prevention services is especially challenging given system-wide change. The communication revolution and recent advances in science have been accompanied by new ways of financing, organizing, and delivering health services at a pitch not realized since the advent of Medicare and Medicaid. Public health professionals in administration and financing also need to play key roles in informing policy that ensures coverage and access for all.

(e) The Evolution to Competency-Based Education

The proliferation of competency statements, the existing variation in core requirements across the schools, and, most especially, the changes occurring in the field have prompted the deans of the 31 accredited graduate schools of public health, as mentioned before, to revisit the issue of master's level public health competence. A current aim of the ongoing ASPH competency development project is to ensure that

M.P.H. graduates are prepared to meet the challenges of practice in the new century. The ASPH Education Committee, as charged by the deans and supported by the membership, is attempting first to recognize the significant changes in the composition and expectations of our students, the demands of employers for more well-rounded students, the scrutiny of the public regarding the benefits of higher education, the challenges that science provokes, and the needs of communities to be served, and, in light of that recognition, to recommend areas of core competence that should be achieved by the M.P.H. curriculum.

The need to effectively measure academic public health performance is exigent and a long-standing vacuum in whole-person, population based funding in research that prevents disease and disability has distressed the health of academia. Performance measurement systems, which measure public health practice as defined by the Essential Public Health Services, aim to provide information to advocate for public health at state and local levels, shape policy decisions, and target resources to ultimately improve the health of the public. Performance measures represent one movement that resounds in many schools of public health that will lead to improvements in training, curricula, and research; enhance accountability and highlight best practices; as well as increase the science base for practice-based research, teaching, and service in SPHs.

(f) Credentialing the Public Health Workforce

As weaknesses in the public health infrastructure have become more obvious, the need to certify and credential the public workforce has grown. The American Public Health Association (APHA) and ASPH have been exploring options for credentialing the workforce with the practice community and plan to collaborate with key practice organizations in developing a system for credentialing public health workers. It is expected that the emerging credential for public health will contribute towards professionalization of the workforce, increase the visibility of public health practice, and assisting in assuring that public health meets the needs of the nation.

02/28/02

Association of State and Territorial Health Officials Answers for the IOM Study on Educating Public Health Professionals for the 21st Century

1. Why would your organization or the members of your organization consider hiring someone with a public health education?

The Association of State and Territorial Health Officials (ASTHO) is the national non-profit organization representing the state and territorial public health agencies of the United States, the U.S. Territories, and the District of Columbia. ASTHO's members, the chief health officials of these jurisdictions, are dedicated to formulating and influencing sound public health policy, and to assuring excellence in state-based public health practice.

A stable and effective public health infrastructure, including sufficient numbers of appropriately trained health professionals distributed to provide appropriate public health services to all populations, is essential to ensure development of sound public health policy and excellence in public health practice. A public health education experience can provide persons who propose to engage in the practice of public health with valuable skills and perspectives critical to a full appreciation of their discipline. Individuals with these critical skills and perspectives are sought because they are likely to be successful in advancing the mission and goals of a public health agency.

2. What is the minimum knowledge you or your organization's members expect from someone with a public health education?

ASTHO supports the use of the three core functions—assessment, assurance, and policy development—as previously described by the Institute of Medicine, and the 10 essential services to improve the practice of public health. ASTHO and its members also acknowledge that it is unlikely that all of our nation's state and local health departments will be fully staffed by persons with a master's degree in public health. With the richness of the various disciplines that comprise the public health workforce, it is important to consider the concept of a public health education in its broadest construct and not limited to graduate academic programs. It is more productive at this time to consider the concept of levels or stages of minimum knowledge in public health, linked to progressively broader and more complex competencies. If considered in this manner, the core competencies for public health professionals published by The Council on Linkages Between Academia and Public Health Practice are one example of how the minimum knowledge base can be described. For example, to improve the overall practice of public health ASTHO supports the use of assessment, planning and evaluation; information for health status monitoring and improvement; *Healthy People 2010* objectives with their leading health indicators and community health status profiles; bioterrorism and emergency preparedness; health data, health data systems; and the capacity of the state and local public health information infrastructure to appropriately measure population health status. Individual members of the public health workforce should be well trained in the specific skills of their discipline; they should have opportunities for ongoing learning; and they should have the skills required to be effective team members in our evolving health care system.

3.   What do you or your organization's members view as the most important areas for educating public health professionals?

Within the construct of levels or stages of public health knowledge and competencies, there is a need to establish realistic competency expectations for each level/stage of "public health education." Such a model encompasses the skills, knowledge, and attitudes necessary for health professionals without a formal public health degree working in a public health practice setting at one end of the continuum (i.e., professional education in a related field such as medicine, nursing, or social work) to those with advanced degrees in public health working in either practice or academic settings (i.e., doctoral education in public health) at the other end of the continuum. The levels or stages of public health education also must consider the competencies that need to be transmitted via continuing education methods for the current public health workforce (both with and without advanced degrees in public health) as well as the competencies of newly prepared public health practitioners graduating from public health graduate programs. While discipline specific competencies remain necessary for specialized roles within public health, promoting the use of the three core functions and the 10 essential services to improve the practice of public health is the keystone upon which all educational plans must be built. Academic public health programs must focus their attention on preparing their graduates for employment in public health practice settings. This has to involve on-going collaboration with the practice community as curricula are developed.

It is critically important that ways be found to build upon the existing public health infrastructure by measuring and continuously improving capacity, resources, skills, partnerships, and activities promoting a national public health performance standards program. This necessitates the availability of a network of appropriate training programs for the continuing education of the existing public health workforce as well as the availability of appropriate educational programs for the preparation of those newly entering the field of public health. Coordination and collaboration with the HRSA Public Health Training Centers and the CDC Centers for Public Health Preparedness is essential. The current geographic disparities in educational opportunities must be addressed in the process and ways to promote the equitable distribution of professionals prepared to practice in public health setting must be found.

4. What do you or your organization's members see as the strengths and challenges facing public health education today?

Compared to earlier eras, public health education today has been strengthened by the development of greater rigor in the underlying academic disciplines, accompanied by considerable expansion of the research (theory) basis of public health practice. Federal agencies such as HRSA, CDC, and NIH have provided important support for this development. In addition, important recent efforts such as the Public Health Workforce Development Collaborative and the Council on Linkages Between Academia and Public Health Practice have improved the coordination between most of the critical entities involved in public health workforce development.

The key challenge facing public health education today is reconciliation of the academic environment in which most public health education takes place with the practice environment for which students are destined. Academic public health institutions and their faculty have a strong and entirely appropriate interest in research; the financial environment of American academic institutions reinforces that focus. All too often, the result of this focus is delivery of public health education that better addresses academic and research issues than the realities of public health practice. Public health education is challenged, as a number of health professions are challenged, to deliver an educational program that is simultaneously academically rigorous and practice oriented. Further, there remains a need to maximize investments in public health workforce training resources and endeavors and to ensure that those in need of training have access to appropriate and high quality offerings. Again, the workforce development efforts in the states as well as the HRSA and CDC Centers and the state/regional/national leadership institutes must be part of the public health training system. The distribution of well-trained and qualified public and personal health service providers, at all levels of the workforce continuum, remains an issue of grave concern to state health agencies and to many special populations in need of providers sensitive to their unique physical, emotional, spiritual, and cultural needs.

5.   What, in your opinion, are changes that might occur in the next 10 years that will call for new skills/knowledge to be added to public health professional training?

Public health agencies, both state and local, must become more successful in fostering systematic public health responses to population health needs. The movement of public health agencies away from a central role as "health care centers for the poor" will probably continue and accelerate over the coming decade. At the same time, the need for public health activities to provide bridging and wrap-around services, to build community coalitions, to maintain and enhance surveillance and assessment activities, and to bring forward creative policy solutions to the health needs of our populations continues. The academic public health profession and public health practice must assure their states and communities understand the critical need and value of such activities. Much of the past support for these critical activities has "slipstreamed" funding for personal health care services delivered by public health agencies. As the health care role of public health changes, public health agencies face a fundamental challenge to "sell" their residual roles to the public and policymakers who have been willing to pay for public health as a welfare function but have not demonstrated a similar willingness to pay for population directed public health services. Public health agencies will need leaders and staff who have the understanding and skills to market the population role that will become more central for public health agencies in the coming decade.

Bioterrorism response and emergency preparedness have heightened awareness of the public safety role of public health and focused attention on some of the functions noted above. Even as we move to strengthen capacity to fulfill the public health role in responding to bioterrorism, we must be careful that such moves not distort the underlying focus of public health on continuous improvement of the health of the public but rather serve to strengthen the infrastructure that is so vital to our success.

03/01/02

Centers for Disease Control Answers for the IOM Study on Educating Public Health Professionals for the 21st Century

INTRODUCTION

The Centers for Disease Control and Prevention has a 50-year tradition of providing and supporting education and training for public health professionals. We applaud the work of the Institute of Medicine Committee on Educating Public Health Professionals for the 21st century and appreciate the opportunity to comment on the questions you posed for consideration.

QUESTIONS:

1.   Why would your organization or the members of your organization consider hiring someone with a public health education?

Public health education (IOM) context: *"We're trying to be fairly inclusive when talking about public health education but we will be focusing on CEPH accredited schools of public health and accredited M.P.H. programs."* L. Hernandez (IOM)

CDC Response:

The mission of the CDC is to promote health and quality of life by preventing and controlling disease, injury, and disability. The accomplishment of the mission is predicated on the following agency strengths:

- prevention strategies based on sound scientific knowledge,
- leadership and technologic capabilities of state and local health organizations and integration of those capabilities with private health organizations,
  - trained public health workers and leaders,
  - ability to serve a diverse population with a diverse workforce.

Trained public health workers are a fundamental capacity for our organization. As an employer, CDC seeks ways to enhance the skills of its employees through its Corporate University and other opportunities for advance studies in public health. For additional information about the Corporate University, contact Sylvia Bell or Carol Higbee, Human Resources Management Office at 770-488-1856. Dale Indergaard at 770-488-1756 can provide specific statistics on fellowships, internships, and job descriptions.

2.   What is the minimum knowledge you or your organization's members expect from someone with a public health education?

For individual with M.P.H. or equivalent from a CEPH accredited program, the agency would anticipate minimum knowledge in:*

1. Biostatistics — collection, storage, retrieval, analysis and interpretation of health data; design and analysis of health-related surveys and experiments; and concepts and practice of statistical data analysis.
2. Epidemiology — distributions and determinants of disease, disabilities and death in human populations; the characteristics and dynamics of human populations; and the natural history of disease and the biologic basis of health.
3. Environmental health sciences — environmental factors including biological, physical, and chemical factors that affect the health of a community.
4. Health services administration — planning, organization, administration, management, evaluation, and policy analysis of health programs.
5. Social and behavioral sciences — concepts and methods of social and behavioral sciences relevant to the identification and the solution of public health problems.

3.   What do you or your organization's members see as the most important areas for educating public health professionals?

In the *CDC/ATSDR Strategic Plan for Public Health Workforce Development* (1999), developed in collaboration with a broad range of academic and practice community partners, task force members articulated three curriculum levels required for the public health workforce: basic, cross-cutting, and discipline-specific (technical/categorical). Basic or "Public Health 101" —provides an overview of public health, history, core values, functions, essential services, and other content as required by local area need, organizational focus, and individual role/responsibility. Cross-cutting—designed to develop core competency skills from basic through intermediate and advanced as required by role/responsibility and career path;

The recently published Council on Linkages document "Core Competencies for Public Health Professionals" (April 2001) provides detailed

---

*From CEPH program accreditation standards.

descriptions of cross-cutting competencies needed to assure that public health agencies have a workforce prepared to deliver essential public health services. The eight domains listed include: analytic assessment skills, basic public health sciences, cultural competency, communication skills, community dimensions of practice, financial planning and management skills, leadership and systems thinking, and policy/program planning. (Additional information is available at http://www.Training Finder.org/competencies.)

Specific emerging needs include: informatics, genomics, public health systems, behavioral/social sciences, health/risk communications, bioterrorism/emergency/disaster preparedness, injury prevention and control, environmental health, evaluation, and ethics. Experience in state or local public health provides a context for policy and practice and is an important component of public health education.

4. What do you or your organization's members see as the strengths and challenges facing public health education today?

Strengths

- Increase in CEPH accredited schools of public health, graduate programs in community health, and graduate programs in community health/preventive medicine;
- Increased access to learning through distance education and certificate programs (meeting needs of adult learners);
- Increased recognition of the importance of public health by general public and political leaders.

Challenges

- Accredited programs are not always accessible;
- Expanding the pipeline into public health, enhancing learning opportunities and workforce diversity;
- Lack of partnership with the practice community in training/education development, implementation and evaluation;
- Growth of non-CEPH accredited programs; graduates enter workforce with various levels of preparation in basic public health science;
- Balancing research and education and service mission (rewarding faculty for practice-focused activities);
- No consistent approach to enumeration of the public health workforce; forecasting personnel needs or related training requirements is limited;

- National consensus on basic and cross-cutting competencies does not yet exist;
  - An integrated delivery system for life-long learning does not exist;
  - Inadequate incentives for participation in training and continuing education;
  - Financing of workforce training and continuing education is hampered by the absence of a coherent policy framework and strategies for funding these activities.

Additional Comments

The public health workforce is multidisciplinary. Individuals enter the field of practice from a broad range of undergraduate and graduate preparation programs. Entry to practice for specific clinical areas such as medicine, nursing, dentistry, etc., is licensed. There is no systematic approach to assure ongoing competency in public health practice through certification, credentialing, or a systematic approach to life long learning opportunities for front line public health professionals. The *CDC/ATSDR Strategic Plan for Public Health Workforce Development* and complementary *Global and National Implementation Plan for Public Health Workforce Development* proposes a flexible three-tiered framework for addressing this complex issue. Expert panel members envisioned a framework with agreement on three levels of certification: basic, discipline-specific and integrator/leader.

- **basic** or orientation level would be available for every public health practitioner completing a "core" practice-focused curriculum (awareness level learning experience);
  - **discipline-specific** certification would result from strengthening public health competencies within existing certification systems (i.e., medical specialty boards; other licensing bodies);
  - **integrator/leader** level would address the unique competencies required of public health system leaders.

Incentives (individual or organizational) should function synergistically within the public health system to enhance capacity to perform essential services and ultimately impact health outcomes. Therefore, the consequences of any incentive system(s) must be carefully considered and strategies developed to reinforce positive effects and ameliorate unintended negative effects.

5.   What, in your opinion, are the changes that might occur in the next 10 years that will call for new skills/knowledge to be added to public health professional training?

- advances in understanding of the human genome may transform medical practice and in turn significantly change public health practice (e.g., treatments for chronic diseases, birth defects, vaccines, environment and health . . .);
- changing demographics—focus on geriatrics and enriched understanding of cultural dimension of health; global health issues;
- increased understanding of environmental influences on health;
- occupational and environmental health;
- informatics and information technology—adaptation and use of a broad range of technology in public health practice;
- emerging infections/drug resistance;
- availability of incentives to pursue life long learning;
- learning technologies will change the way professional education is obtained (advance distance learning);
- advances in neuroscience—mental health;
- health and spirituality—mind/body connection; alternative/complementary medicine; stress and health.

National Association of County and City Health Officials Answers for the IOM Study on Educating Public Health Professionals for the 21st Century

1. Why would your organization or the members of your organization consider hiring someone with a public health education?

The work of NACCHO is directed at improving and supporting the practice of public health at the local level. A candidate for hiring that brings either local experience or a good grasp of public health as obtained through a course of education/training is fairly well prepared to begin contributing to NACCHO's work. Without that, we must spend time and effort training new hires.

2.   What is the minimum knowledge you or your organization's members expect from someone with a public health education?

We rarely hire someone with a PH education who doesn't have an M.P.H. We expect someone with an M.P.H. to have a broad grasp of public health principles, history, and understanding of the general programs and methods used in the field, and a good grasp of the terminology. We have hired staff with M.P.A.s, M.B.A.s, Ph.D.s, and other advanced degrees outside public health and have had good luck with most. They do, however, require a little more time up front with orientation and vocabulary building. I also need to add here that someone with an average to very good public health education is NOT fully prepared for practice, and is not fully prepared to work at NACCHO. Nearly all lack exposure to community dynamics and the varying challenges that practitioners experience daily. Experience, even if through on-the-job exposure, is absolutely essential. We try to rotate all of our staff through local health departments for a substantial exposure.

3.   What do you or your organization's members view as the most important areas for educating public health professionals?

More and more we are hearing that public health professionals need more training in leadership, management, community organization, communications, and trans-disciplinary orientation (e.g., orientation to city planning, law enforcement, etc.) While a good grounding in the basic public health sciences is important for some staff in a public health organization (e.g., biostat, epidemiology), local health officials indicate that more if not all staff need expertise in the other five areas mentioned.

4. What do you or your organization's members see as the strengths and challenges facing public health education today?

The strengths are that there are alternatives (schools and programs), and that they are fairly widely available. Many offer midcareer courses of study.

The challenges seem to be significant and daunting: while some gains have been made, there continues to be a disconnect between public health academia and practice. Most M.P.H. students (estimated at 80 percent by ASPH) do not pursue a career in public health. Most schools and programs appear to have little interest in addressing the training needs of public health practitioners (outside of a course of study leading to a degree). There is little connection between the course of study and practical experience opportunities in most schools, and most schools do NOT utilize the practice expertise of practitioners in shared teaching arrangements. Few academicians venture out into practice to learn from and contribute to practice. Research conducted by schools of public health is seldom practice oriented, and where it is, there is often very poor translation to and connection between practice research findings and practice.

5. What, in your opinion, are changes that might occur in the next 10 years that will call for new skills/knowledge to be added to public health professional training?

Infrastructure is being built at the state and local level as an outcome of bioterrorism and resultant funding. The growing staff component of tomorrow's health departments will require short courses in the public health sciences, as well as training in a variety of areas. As mentioned above, schools of public health have a very poor track record of addressing such needs, and often aren't even qualified to address practice needs. I believe schools should begin moving capacity to address this building need. Several strategies should be considered, including:

• including local and state public health practitioners as part of faculty;
• conducting research regarding where current public health professionals have been trained, where they obtain on-going professional training, where they would like to get training, barriers to training and education, etc.;
• granting access to libraries and other resources of the schools for public health practitioners in the area;

- pursuing "practical" research in state and local public health settings;
- increasing responsibility/focus on continuing education for public health professionals;
- engaging public health faculty in undergraduate training of professions which work with or are hired by public health agencies, such as nursing, environmental health;
- developing stronger linkages during training between academic work and field practice.

Public Health Foundation Answers for the IOM Study on Educating Public Health Professionals for the 21st Century

1. Why would your organization or the members of your organization consider hiring someone with a public health education?

While we do not limit our hiring to individuals with a public health degree, the M.P.H. is very attractive to the Public Health Foundation (PHF). We strongly desire well-rounded individuals with knowledge and skills in the basic sciences of public health and research methods. In addition, we value individuals who have practical experience in public health practice and have developed expertise as effective communicators, conveners, and consensus builders. The ideal for us is an individual educated in public health with practical experience and training received in a public health practice setting.

2. What is the minimum knowledge you or your organization's members expect from someone with a public health education?

Our organization looks for people with knowledge and skills in each of the eight domains of the core competencies for public health professionals (adopted by the Council on Linkages Between Academia and Public Health Practice in April 2001). While we do not expect individuals to have skills for each of the competencies (there are over 60), we do expect individuals to have knowledge and skills in each of the eight competency domains. Unfortunately, our expectations often go unmet.

3. What do you or your organization's members view as the most important areas for educating public health professionals?

Education occurs in many ways and in many settings. For this question, we focus on graduate-level education and continuing education of the current workforce.

While graduate-level education typically provides an individual with an excellent understanding of the theories of public health, often times a comprehensive orientation to public health practice does not occur. In addition, much of the graduate-level training is increasingly moving towards specialization. This is resulting in fewer graduates with a well-rounded education. To round out one's education and provide a greater orientation to practice, graduate-level education should include: 1) greater use of case studies; 2) involvement of students in applied research activities; 3) exercises on writing to non-academic audiences for identified purposes; 4) training on finding information and determining its quality; and 5) a greater focus on qualitative analysis.

As in virtually all professions, continuing education also is essential in public health. Many in the current workforce, while extremely skilled in many technical areas, lack a basic understanding of public health concepts, frameworks, and principles, such as the Essential Public Health Services and *Healthy People 2010*. In addition, continuing education is needed in areas such as: 1) understanding, using, and managing information technology; 2) applied research methods; and 3) finding, understanding, and using the scientific evidence in public health.

4.   What do you or your organization's members see as the strengths and challenges facing public health education today?

In schools of public health, there are more practice opportunities today than possibly at any time in the past. This is a major strength of public health education today. In addition, there are more schools of public health and enrollees, resulting in more well-educated graduates in public health. For the current workforce, there also are hundreds of distance learning courses available as well as on-site continuing education opportunities.

One of the greatest challenges facing public health practice education are market forces. Too few graduates of schools of public health end up working in public health practice settings, especially the more traditional state and local health agency settings. Because of this reality, schools may not tailor their curriculum to the needs of governmental public health. For this to change, agencies need to be willing to hire, and appropriately pay, graduates of schools of public health. Otherwise, schools may continue to move away from providing appropriate education for individuals desiring to work in public health agency settings. In addition, Federal support for teaching in public health has become virtually nonexistent. These funds are vital for supporting faculty training and developing much-needed case study materials. Other market forces, such as continued emphasis by funding agencies on basic science research (with little emphasis on public health systems research), results in faculty focusing their research energies on non-practice questions. If students are to develop a greater understanding of applied research techniques and develop an appreciation for evidence-based approaches to public health practice, funding of this type of research is essential.

Another challenge facing public health education is that there are too few courses designed to build knowledge and skills in many of the core public health competencies. For example, there are few courses addressing cultural competence needs and approaches for working with stakeholders.

There are many challenges also facing continuing education for the current public health workforce. While hundreds of distance learning courses have been developed and are available to all public health professionals, there are few, if any, standards to enable a potential student to distinguish a quality course from one of lesser quality. Even when quality courses are identified, often times the employer does not permit time off to take the course or provide the funds necessary for enrolling in the course. Finally, while distance learning and on-site continuing education exist, the most appropriate technologies and adult learning techniques are not fully utilized by the public health profession.

5. What, in your opinion, are changes that might occur in the next 10 years that will call for new skills/knowledge to be added to public health professional training?

The greatest challenge is to meet the current identified needs that have gone unmet for well over a decade already. For many years, experts in public health practice and academia have identified training needs in areas such as: 1) cultural competence; 2) the basics of public health practice; 3) managing contracts; 4) managing information and technology; and 5) accountability and performance management. Needs in these areas are likely to increase throughout this decade and beyond. To more completely understand the current and future education and training needs of the public health workforce, a comprehensive assessment using the core competencies for public health professionals could be conducted that identifies gaps and priority training needs. Other new skill/knowledge needs are likely to be in the areas of genomics, how to identify and use the growing body of scientific evidence that can guide the practice of public health, and strategies for integrating the aging population into public health programs.

Appendix D

The Education of Public Health Professionals in the 20th Century

Elizabeth Fee

PREAMBLE

Over the past 50 years or more, many reports and conference proceedings have discussed the nation's system of public health education. In general, these tend to deplore the general state of public health education and the inadequate preparation of the public health "workforce." Recently, Kristine Gebbie crisply summed up the contemporary state of the discussion in her editorial, "The Public Health Workforce: Key to Public Health Infrastructure."[1] A longer version of the argument[2] joins a series of recent publications and manifestos on the problems of public health education.[3, 4] These in turn appear to derive some of their general framework from the rather unflattering view of public health encapsulated in the Institute of Medicine's report of 1988 on *The Future of Public Health*.[5] Briefly character-

---

[1] Kristine M. Gebbie, The Public Health Workforce: Key to Public Health Infrastructure, *American Journal of Public Health*, 89, 1999: 660–661.

[2] Gebbie K, Hwang I. *Preparing Currently Employed Public Health Professionals for Changes in the Health System*. New York: Columbia University School of Nursing; 1998.

[3] Public Health Functions Project, *The Public Health Workforce: An Agenda for the 21st Century*. U.S. Department of Health and Human Services, Washington, D.C.: 1998. This document calls for "a reassessment and a retooling of the entire public health education and training enterprise"(p. 7), with lots of "partnerships," "collaborations," and "stakeholder groups" measuring "performance-based competencies."

[4] Andrew A. Sorenson and Ronald G. Bialek, *The Public Health Faculty/Agency Forum: Linking Graduate Education and Practice—Final Report*. Gainesville, Fl: University of Florida Press; 1993.

[5] Institute of Medicine, *The Future of Public Health*. Washington, DC: National Academy Press; 1988.

ized, these various analyses assert that public health departments are poorly staffed, and that many of the people working in them lack the specific skills, qualifications, and abilities they need to fulfill their responsibilities of protecting the public health. The faculty members of public health schools, for their part, are busy doing research, and training students to do research, but they are failing to turn out the highly educated labor pool needed to adequately staff the public health departments of the future. Phrased another way, the "theory" of public health as taught in the academy does not cohere tightly to its "practice" as performed in state and local health departments. Public health "leadership" is said to be needed to connect the fragmented pieces by taking the knowledge produced in the schools and applying it in the "laboratory" of people's lives.

Within schools of public health, most faculty members are scientists and researchers with a Ph.D. degree. Few have any work experience outside of academia, much less in city or state health departments. Not surprisingly, they have little interest in becoming engaged with the practical work of public health agencies. Many, especially in the laboratory-centered disciplines, have little knowledge of, or interest in, politics or policy, or they regard politics as merely some distasteful contaminant of an otherwise orderly search for knowledge. Even social and behavioral scientists are often more interested in their statistical methodologies than with the messy arts of organization, advocacy, and policy-making. They shy away from the popular media, television cameras, news magazines, street demonstrations—among the various modes of informing, shaping, and challenging public opinion—as perhaps undignified and definitely distracting. Nor are they often to be found in the schools, clinics, churches, and community organizations of the decaying sections of the cities in which they work.

From the point of view of the faculty of public health schools and programs, there is little time for the multiplicity of things they are already being pressured to do. To be required to raise the best part of one's own salary, and to write grants to cover research assistants, secretaries, students, equipment, or other research needs, focuses the mind admirably. All other activities become luxuries. To be successful in the research funding world requires associated and time-consuming commitments: to read the work of one's colleagues, to review other people's grant applications, to publish on a regular basis, to participate in academic and professional meetings, to have pieces of one's time scattered across other people's projects in case one's own project lacks sufficient funding. None of this allows much leisure for intellectual or political activities that are not directly related to the research agenda, such as exploring the messy world of community organizations or writing for popular, as opposed to scientific, journals. It is only on rare occasions and more or less by accident that schools of public health harbor public intellectuals or effective public advocates for the public's health.

If schools of public health have become mainly research institutes, where students learn the art of preparing grant proposals and writing scientific articles, what about the local departments of public health? In general, these are staffed by people with little public health training—people who learn the processes and problems of public health on the job. Some have scientific, medical, nursing, or engineering degrees that may be relevant to their work but the matching of credentials to tasks is often haphazard. Certainly, there is no assumption that all members of a local health department will be graduates of an accredited school of public health. Salaries in public health are low and political pressures are often strong; many public health departments survive in a more or less permanent state of crisis, coping with the last budget cut and waiting for the next one. Their contact with the schools of public health is likely to be sporadic—a lecture series here and there, an occasional joint project.

If there is indeed something lacking in the structure and processes of public health education, then, from the historian's perspective, it is useful to find out when the problem started. Has it always been thus? How did this state of things come to pass? What forces are responsible for the peculiar disjuncture between schools of public health and the departments of public health where the work of public health gets done? In order to explore these questions, we need to examine the two general phases of public health education in America: the phase of private funding by the great philanthropies when independent schools of public health were first created and second, the period of federal and state funding. Although there is overlap between these two phases, it seems reasonable to date the first as 1914–1939, and the second as 1935 to the present. As part of phase two were the wartime programs in public health funded by the armed services.

After the war, as in other sectors of the economy, there was a long era of postwar expansion, with smaller bumps and recessions along the way. Overall, funding for public health education has been on an upward trajectory but the development has been uneven; wavelike patterns of expansion and retrenchment make for instability and great difficulty in planning. If health departments have often lurched from crisis to crisis, schools of public health have accustomed themselves to an often erratic funding cycle, with sudden infusions of funds for special areas of concentration, political shifts and cutbacks, and the giving and taking away again of grants and training funds. The miracle of it all is that so many excellent and talented students pass through, are educated, and receive credentials, before emerging into the intersecting worlds of government agencies, voluntary associations, foundations, academia, international organizations, and managed care companies.

THE FOUNDING OF SCHOOLS OF PUBLIC HEALTH

The first independent schools of public health in the United States were funded and nurtured by the Rockefeller Foundation. Rockefeller philanthropies were by far the largest and most important in terms of their influence on public health education, so I will focus on them here, but it is notable that other foundations, such as Commonwealth, Kellogg, and Milbank, were also extremely involved in and supportive of public health education during the interwar years. Not until 1935 did the federal government provide any significant level of funding for public health education.

To set the context for the recurring struggles over public health education, it may be helpful to note that medical schools had proliferated throughout the 19th century because they were economically advantageous to both faculty and students. A few faculty members could get together, create a medical school, and charge tuition; assuming the fees were not too high, nor the entrance requirements too strict, the students would come. Then as now, medical students were making a wise investment in their future earnings. Schools of nursing, by contrast, were created by hospitals that needed a well-trained and well-behaved labor force to staff their wards; the hospitals thus had an economic interest in creating their own diploma schools. Once the nursing profession was more fully established, universities found that women students (or their families) were willing to pay tuition as an investment in a respected female career. In the case of public health, however, by the later 19th century, when cities and states were calling for public health officers, there were no established career patterns. Public health leaders were generally people like Hermann Biggs or Josephine Baker—physicians who, with lucrative private medical practices on the side, could devote themselves to the public's health as a largely voluntary activity. The rank and file of public health officers were simply practicing physicians who could be called out in times of crisis to assist in coping with epidemic diseases, but who were otherwise fully involved in caring for their own patients. Municipalities employed a variety of health inspectors and street cleaners but these were largely untrained and often unreliable workers, many of whom obtained their positions through political patronage.

It was thus the leaders of the Rockefeller philanthropies who, in the early 20th century, set themselves the task of creating a public health profession. The Rockefeller officers became involved in public health education because of their experience with the hookworm eradication campaign in the southern United States. The hookworm eradication campaign was part of a massive program to modernize the South—besides building railroads and factories, the representatives of northern capital would raise the productivity of the rural southern workforce by eliminating the "germ of laziness."[6] This was a perfectly logical approach because hookworm infestation produces anemia and thus decreases the population's ability to work; a healthier workforce would indeed be more productive.

Members of the Rockefeller Sanitary Commission's staff had initially assumed that they could rely on public health officers in the southern states to help carry out their program. But to their distress, they found these part-time health officers displayed little interest in or dedication to the task. Rural southern physicians disliked the northern Yankees, resented being ordered about, and generally refused to believe that hookworm was a serious problem. Wickliffe Rose, the architect and organizer of the Rockefeller Sanitary Commission, came to believe that a new profession was needed—separate from medicine—composed of men and women who would devote their whole careers to the control of disease. Rose insisted that there must be two professions: medicine, for treating disease at an individual level, and public health, for controlling disease and promoting health at a population level.

Rose turned to Abraham Flexner whose "Flexner Report" of 1910 had been central to the reorganization of American medical education.[7] Flexner was then head of the General Education Board, the Rockefeller organization responsible for education programs. Flexner was involved in a struggle to make medical school professors "full-time" faculty—to separate teaching and research from private practice so that professors would be able to devote their entire attention to their academic pursuits. To Rose, the problem of part-time health officers appeared in a similar light: public health practitioners should be "full-time" so that they would devote their whole attention to the needs of public health and not be distracted by the demands of private practice.

Flexner found that Rose's concerns were widely shared by prominent leaders in public health. Indeed, the Massachusetts Institute of Technology and Harvard University had already put together an impressive curriculum for training health officers in communicable diseases, sanitary engineering, preventive medicine, demography, public health administration, sanitary biology, and sanitary chemistry.[8] Students generally entered with professional degrees—they could be engineers or physicians—and completed a two or three year course of additional study before receiving a certificate in public health. The combined program graduated a small number of highly-trained health officers each year.

---

[6] John Ettling, *The Germ of Laziness: Rockefeller Philanthropy and Public Health in the New South.* Cambridge: Harvard University Press, 1981.

[7] Abraham Flexner, *Medical Education in the United States and Canada.* Bulletin No. 4. New York: Carnegie Endowment for the Advancement of Teaching, 1910.

[8] Jean Alonzo Curran, *Founders of the Harvard School of Public Health with Biographical Notes, 1909–1946.* New York: Josiah Macy, Jr., Foundation, 1970.

Hearing about the interest of the General Education Board, and hoping for some of the Rockefeller largesse, several universities submitted competing proposals for a school of public health. Harvard University naturally thought that the project could best be entrusted to them, and had in mind an expanded School for Health Officers. Charles-Edward A. Winslow, however, argued in favor of a school in New York City that would focus on training public health nurses, sanitary inspectors, and health officers for small towns—the rank and file of the profession, not just the most highly educated elite. Wickliffe Rose agreed that one or two schools could be established and asked Abraham Flexner to organize a planning conference for October 1914.[9]

Columbia University now submitted a plan for a school—combining medical, engineering, and social science courses—to be established in New York. The Columbia plan especially emphasized the social and political sciences, in contrast to the more usual emphasis upon biological sciences and sanitary engineering. In the discussions that followed, three competing conceptions of public health emerged: the engineering or environmental approach, the sociopolitical, and the biomedical. In the end, the biomedical approach would dominate, with sociopolitical and environmental concerns relegated to a very subsidiary role.

Wickliffe Rose asked Abraham Flexner to consult with medical school professors, members of the newly formed United States Public Health Service, the medical departments of the army and navy, state and city health departments, registrars of vital statistics, representatives of life insurance companies, and health managers of large industries. Flexner, however, preferred to rely on the advice of a few trusted friends and never consulted most of these varied experts. Instead, he brought together a group of 20: 11 public health representatives and 9 Rockefeller trustees and officers for a one-day meeting on October 16, 1914. The decisions made during that conference would shape public health education for the next 25 years.

First was the question of the types of practitioners for whom training was needed. Hermann Biggs, the health commissioner of New York state, declared that there were essentially three classes of public health officers. The "health officials of the first class," were those with executive authority such as city and state health commissioners. The health officials of the "second class" were the technical experts in specific fields: bacteriologists, statisticians, engineers, chemists, and epidemiologists who would run health department programs and conduct research. The "third class," the "subordinates" or "actual field workers," were the local health officials,

---

[9] These matters are discussed in greater detail in Elizabeth Fee, *Disease and Discovery: A History of the Johns Hopkins School of Hygiene and Public Health, 1916–1939*. Baltimore: The Johns Hopkins University Press, 1987, esp. 26–56.

factory and food inspectors, and public health nurses. Members of this last and most numerous group would be the "foot soldiers" in the war against disease.

The most difficult question was whether the "first class" officials had to be medical men. If public health were to become a full-time career, was it reasonable to suppose that physicians would be willing to give up their independence to become salaried employees? As a consequence of the Flexner reforms in medical education, physicians' incomes were rising sharply, so it was hardly a propitious time to expect a large influx of doctors into public health. But William Henry Welch of Johns Hopkins brushed these concerns aside, stating—as it would turn out, with excessive optimism—that physicians would be eager for the "splendid opportunity" of education in public health. Hermann Biggs argued in vain that the requirement of a medical degree was unrealistic, for most of those present at the meeting believed that only medically qualified health officers would be able to gain the cooperation of medical men in the community. Already, the potential for conflict between medical men and public health officers was evident to these experienced observers but the proposed solution—to make public health officers medical men—would prove ineffective. It did not address the real source of the conflict and ignored the looming contradiction between the interests of the majority of the medical profession, engaged in fee-for-service private practice—and a new minority group of salaried public health doctors.

At the October conference, Wickliffe Rose laid out a carefully articulated vision of the future of public health education. At the center he placed a scientific school, well endowed for research. This school would belong to a university but be independent—specifically, it would not be a department of a medical school. Students attending the school would be selected from across the country and its graduates would be carefully placed in strategic positions throughout the United States. This central scientific school would be linked to simpler schools of public health to be established in every state; these state schools would focus on teaching rather than on research. The state schools would in turn be affiliated with medical schools and with state health departments and would offer short training courses for health officers already in the field. Following the pattern of the agricultural extension courses and farm demonstration programs that the Rockefeller Foundation had already used to modernize agriculture in the southern states, they would offer extension services for rural health education.[10] Both central and state schools would teach public education methods and seek to extend public health information to the entire population. The central school would take the whole country as its

---

[10] See Abraham Flexner, *The General Education Board, 1902–1914.* New York: General Education Board, 1915, pp. 18–70.

"field of operations," sending out "an army of workers" to demonstrate the best methods of public health, and bringing back their practical experience to be "assembled and capitalized" at the center of operations.[11]

Rose and Welch were given the task of writing up this draft plan to be mailed to the meeting participants for their criticisms and suggestions. Rose now outlined a memorandum entitled "School of Public Health," and Welch countered—at the last possible minute—with a plan for an "Institute of Hygiene."[12] Because of Welch's perhaps unconscious procrastination, there was no time to circulate this document to the meeting participants before its official presentation to the General Education Board; although Rose himself had not had time to review the draft, it was presented as the "Welch-Rose Report." As I have previously argued, Welch's version of the plan was more oriented to scientific research than was Rose's more practice-oriented model; Welch's version dropped almost all mention of Rose's system of state schools, practical demonstrations, and extension courses.[13] Enthusiastic paragraphs about the need for an army of public health nurses and special inspectors had been eliminated; instead, Welch dwelled happily on the development of "the science of hygiene in all its branches" that would be the focus of the central school of public health. He dropped Rose's phrases about the divergent aims of medicine and public health and instead suggested that the new school of public health should be close to a good teaching hospital.

Some of the participants at the October conference and other public health leaders complained that Welch's version of the report was closer to the German than to the English conception of public health. In other words, the focus on research largely ignored public health practice, administration, public health nursing, and health education. The medical side of public health was emphasized to the virtual exclusion of its social and economic context; no mention was made of the political sciences or of the need to plan for social or economic reforms. Public health was to be biomedical, not social in orientation. Abraham Flexner, who greatly admired Welch, brushed aside all such objections and subtly maneuvered the decision-making process towards Welch's ideas and the selection of Johns Hopkins University as the site of the first endowed school of public health. The Johns Hopkins School of Hygiene and Public Health opened its doors to its first class of students during the influenza epidemic of 1918. Only later did the Rockefeller officials agree to provide funding for other schools of public health, most notably at Harvard and Toronto.

---

[11] Wickliffe Rose, "School of Public Health," May 1915, p. 10. Rockefeller Foundation Archives, Record Group 1.1, Series 200. Rockefeller Archive Center, North Tarrytown, New York.

[12] William Henry Welch, "Institute of Hygiene," May 27, 1915, Rockefeller Foundation Archives, Record Group 1.1, Series 200.

[13] Fee, *Disease and Discovery*, 40-42.

Wickliffe Rose's grand conception of a network of state schools with extension agents fanning out into the countryside, major emphases on public health education, short courses and extension courses to upgrade the skills of health officers in the field, and demonstrations of best practices in public health were not implemented by the Rockefeller Foundation—although much would later come into being albeit in a more haphazard and less carefully planned fashion. For most of the Rockefeller men of that era, it made sense to start at the top, create one or two elite schools of public health, and let the rest flow from the center. Had the emphasis on modernization and increasing worker productivity that had been characteristic themes of the hookworm eradication program been maintained as the central motive and justification for public health campaigns, perhaps other private interests would have helped bankroll the rest of Rose's initial vision. But as history turned out, it would take the crisis of the Depression and the creative responses of the New Deal to impel the next major leap forward in public health education.

The first schools of public health: Johns Hopkins, Harvard, Columbia, and Yale, tended for the most part to follow the model set by the Hopkins school. They were well-endowed private institutions with high admission standards; they favored medical graduates, and often admitted rather distinguished mid-career people already experienced in public health. In the 1920s and early 1930s, the curricula of the schools tended to be heavily weighted toward the laboratory sciences: bacteriology, parasitology, immunology, and what was called "physiological hygiene," along with instruction in epidemiology, vital statistics, and public health administration. The main emphasis was on infectious diseases, with some attention to nutrition (biochemistry), water quality, and occupational hazards. In the 1920s, little was attempted in the way of field practice but this was, perhaps, relatively unimportant as so many of the students were already experienced practitioners. The Rockefeller Foundation gave fellowships to medical graduates around the world who were interested in studying public health, so that from the beginning, the schools tended to have an international flavor. The Foundation would later use these graduates to help establish schools of public health in Brazil, Bulgaria, Canada, Czechoslovakia, England, Hungary, India, Italy, Japan, Norway, the Philippines, Poland, Rumania, Sweden, Turkey, and Yugoslavia.

The Rockefeller Foundation also tried to convince the schools to establish programs of field training. Using the model of medical school education, the students, they argued, should learn to practice in the community much as medical students learned their art in the wards of a hospital. Johns Hopkins under Welch had been reluctant to pay much attention to practical training but in the 1930s, with additional funding from the Rockefeller Foundation, Hopkins did establish the Eastern Health District, consisting of a study population of about 100,000 people living in the neighborhoods around the School of Hygiene. These families were intensively studied through a house-to-house health census every three years; as a local newspaper described the population, "They are, by all odds, the most interrogated, surveyed, investigated, and card-indexed citizens of Baltimore—and probably of the 48 states, Alaska, Hawaii, Puerto Rico, and the Philippines."[14] Many of the Hopkins doctoral students wrote their dissertations on some aspect of the health of this population.

By 1930, the first schools of health were turning out a small number of graduates with a sophisticated scientific education. The schools however were doing little or nothing to turn out the large numbers of public health officers, nurses, and sanitarians needed across the nation. In 1932, the American Public Health Association established a Committee on Professional Education chaired by Waller S. Leathers, Dean of the Vanderbilt Medical School, which included many of the then leading names in public health circles, such as Thomas Parran, W.G. Smillie, Allen Freeman, and Huntington Williams, among others. This committee prepared 20 reports on the educational qualifications of 15 professional specialists, and ultimately distributed some 250,000 copies of these reports.[15] The idea of this very considerable effort was to inform state and local health departments about the types of employees they should be seeking and the kinds of qualifications appropriate for each, with the idea of creating national standards that, if used by the multiplicity of local health departments, could create some degree of uniformity across the nation.

FEDERAL FUNDING FOR PUBLIC HEALTH EDUCATION

A major stimulus to the further development of public health education came in response to the Depression, with the New Deal and the Social Security Act of 1935. The Social Security Act expanded financing of the Public Health Service and provided federal grants to the states to assist them in developing their public health services. Federal and state expenditures for public health actually doubled in the decade of the Depression.

Federal law required each state to establish minimal qualifications for health personnel employed through federal assistance, and recommended at least one year of graduate education at an approved school of public health. For the first time, the federal government provided funds, administered through the states, for public health training. Overall, the states budgeted for more than 1,500 public health trainees, and the existing

---

[14] "Where Doorbells Are Always Ringing," *Evening Sun*, September 13, 1939.
[15] William P. Shepard, "The Professionalization of Public Health," *American Journal of Public Health*, 38, 1948: 145–153.

training programs were soon filled to capacity. As a result of the growing demand for public health credentials, several state universities began new schools or divisions of public health and existing schools of public health expanded their enrollments.

In 1936, the American Public Health Association reported that 10 schools offered public health degrees or certificates requiring at least one year of residence; of these, the largest were Johns Hopkins, Harvard, Columbia, and Michigan.[16] Also offering degrees in public health were the universities of California at Berkeley, Massachusetts Institute of Technology, Minnesota, Pennsylvania, Wayne State, and Yale. By 1938, more than 4,000 people, including about 1,000 doctors, had received some public health training with funds provided by the federal government through the states. The economic difficulties of maintaining a private practice during the Depression had pushed some physicians into public health; others were attracted by the availability of fellowships or by increased social awareness of the plight of the poor and of their need for public health services. In 1939, the federal government allotted over $21 million for public health programs: $8 million for maternal and child health, $9 million for general public health work, and $4 million for venereal disease control.

Of course, many students and health departments desired the most efficient and least time-consuming process of credentialing they could find. The market favored programs that could produce the largest numbers of graduates in the least amount of time. When there were not enough places in schools of public health to supply the need, many colleges and universities opened public health departments and programs, some offering training courses of just a few months' or even a few weeks' duration. Engineering programs turned out sanitary engineers by the score. Summer sessions in public health nursing at Berkeley, Michigan, Minnesota, Columbia, Syracuse, Western Reserve, and several other universities produced over 3,000 graduates annually. These short programs offered a variety of diplomas and certificates in public health; by 1939, 45 institutions were offering 18 different degrees, certificates, and diplomas in public health. Of these 45, 10 were independent schools of public health, 20 were colleges and universities offering programs in public health nursing, and 12 were engineering colleges offering programs in sanitary engineering.

Despite a great expansion of public health training facilities, there were still far from enough graduates to meet the demand. Federal training funds were now allotted to California, Michigan, Minnesota, Vanderbilt, and North Carolina to develop short courses for the rapid training of

---

[16] Committee on Professional Education, "Public Health Degrees and Certificates Granted in 1936," *American Journal of Public Health*, 27, 1937, 1267–1272.

public health personnel. These short courses were recognized as emergency measures until the schools were able to develop more adequate graduate educational programs. Perhaps not surprisingly, the faculty of the founding schools of public health generally disapproved of this rush to short training courses. At Harvard, when the Social Security Act was passed in 1935, the faculty immediately understood that there would be a demand for short courses and decided to resist. They unanimously stated that "short courses should not be instituted or standards lowered, no matter what the situations we are asked to meet."[17] To emphasize their concern about maintaining high academic standards, the faculty promptly raised admission standards.[18]

The tremendous push in the late 1930s toward training larger numbers of public health practitioners was also a push toward practical training programs rather than research. Public health departments wanted personnel with one year of public health education: typically, the M.P.H. generalist degree. If they could not attract public health practitioners with this credential, they settled for a person with a few months of public health training. Ideally, they also wanted people who understood practical public health issues rather than scientific specialists with research degrees. Thus, public health education in the 1930s tended to be practically oriented, with considerable emphasis on fields such as public health administration, health education, public health nursing, vital statistics, venereal disease control, and community health services. In this period, too, many schools developed field training programs in local communities where their students could get a taste of the practical world of public health and a preparation for their roles within local health departments. The 1930s were thus the prime years of community-based public health education.

In 1939, the Rockefeller Foundation decided to evaluate the status and future of public health education. The Scientific Directors of the International Health Division selected Thomas Parran, the Surgeon General, and Livingston Farrand, recently retired President of Cornell University, to study the schools of public health in the United States and Canada.[19] Parran and Farrand estimated that about 300 public health physicians and between 2,000 and 4,000 public health nurses would be needed each year to staff public health departments. They also noted an increasing demand for sanitary engineers, epidemiologists, statisticians, and other types of

---

[17] Minutes of the Faculty of Public Health, November 8, 1935, as cited in Curran, *Founders of the Harvard School of Public Health*, p. 56.

[18] *Ibid.*, p. 58.

[19] Thomas Parran and Livingston Farrand, "Report to the Rockefeller Foundation on the Education of Public Health Personnel," October 28, 1939. Rockefeller Foundation Archives, Record Group 1.1, Series 200.

specialists. Parran and Farrand recommended increased support for the schools of public health at Hopkins, Harvard, and Toronto, mainly to sustain research in the core public health disciplines. They also recommended that regional schools of public health be established in the West (suggesting California at Berkeley), the Midwest (Michigan), and the South (Vanderbilt). Such regional schools, they emphasized, should be oriented to practical training rather than to research.

THE WAR YEARS

Not surprisingly, the proliferation of short training programs continued throughout the war years. The armed services wanted physicians, nurses, and sanitarians with at least a minimal amount of training in tropical diseases, parasitology, venereal disease control, environmental sanitation, and a variety of infectious diseases. For the burgeoning industrial production areas at home, industrial hygiene was in demand; for areas with military encampments, sanitary engineering and malaria control were very urgent concerns. In this period, the Center for Controlling Malaria in the War Areas, the forerunner of the Centers for Disease Control and Prevention, was created. Schools of public health and public health training programs changed their educational programs to meet the various needs of the armed services as rapid training programs turned out large numbers of health professionals with a smattering of specialized education in high-priority fields. The research-oriented schools of public health, such as Hopkins and Harvard, maintained their research programs largely by recruiting foreign students—many of them from Latin America—to staff their laboratory and field programs; in those years, Johns Hopkins was said to resemble an outpost of Latin America. The North American students all wanted quick training programs before going to their war posts at home and abroad.

Deans of the leading schools of public health were no doubt anxious about the future direction of public health education—were all these short training programs going to threaten the long-term standards and standing of the best public health education? In 1941, representatives from Columbia, Harvard, Johns Hopkins, Michigan, North Carolina, Toronto, and Yale met to organize the Association of Schools of Public Health, "to promote and improve the graduate education and training of . . . professional personnel for service in public health." The representatives clearly disapproved of many of the new rapid training programs and limited membership in the Association to schools giving graduate degrees. They argued the need for an accreditation mechanism to establish standards of public health education but realized that this goal would have to wait until after the war. The Association had no formal authority over licensing—there has never been any clear agreement over public health credentials—but it claimed a certain moral authority in representing the most highly developed schools of public health.

THE POST-WAR YEARS: TOWARD ACCREDITATION

In 1946, the Committee on Professional Education of the American Public Health Association took over the job of monitoring the standards of public health education. William Shepard, then Third Vice-President of the Metropolitan Life Insurance Company, energetically chaired the committee. Shepard complained about profit-making public health training courses of dubious quality; at least one school was offering public health degrees by correspondence, its "faculty" consisting of several authors of leading texts on public health who were entirely unaware of their "appointment."[20] At least a dozen universities were in the process of establishing schools of public health, some of them with no new faculty— merely using existing faculty as part-time teachers. Proprietary schools, complained Shepard, constituted a "dark period" in the development of a profession—marking the moment when demand for trained people exceeded supply. Given the large demand for public health personnel and the relatively sparse supply, the APHA Committee saw its task in part as differentiating between good and poor candidates and as stemming the tide of poorly-trained "incompetents."

The Committee on Professional Education also created a plan for the accreditation of schools of public health, financed in its earliest years by the Commonwealth Foundation. Thanks to studies by Haven Emerson and Martha Luginbuhl,[21] the Association was able to estimate how many full-time public health personnel were needed in the nation, the replacement rate of existing public health officers, and therefore the number of schools of public health that were really needed—Shepard estimated in 1946 that between 5 and 10 additional schools of public health would be necessary to provide the public health workforce for the nation.

The difficulty with instituting a system of licensing and credentialing was the low salaries involved in most public health positions. With the war and the depression behind, public health positions were failing to attract the most highly-qualified candidates. Physicians, in particular, showed little enthusiasm for public health appointments. The attractions of private and hospital practice far outpaced the appeal of public health agencies. There seemed little point in attempting to impose any form of licensing when the number of jobs so outstripped the number of available candidates, and public health positions for the most part were regarded

---

[20] Shepard, "Professionalization," p. 149.

[21] Haven Emerson and Martha Luginbuhl, *Local Health Units for the Nation*. New York: The Commonwealth Fund, 1945.

as financially undesirable. The Committee's answer to this structural problem was to urge "a comprehensive public relations program under expert direction," which would lead to increased public recognition and thus, perhaps, to higher salaries.

With funding from the U.S. Public Health Service, the Committee now set up a kind of public health employment agency in an attempt to match vacant positions in public health with job candidates. In 1947, the "Vocational Counseling and Placement Service" listed some 688 available public health positions and 164 candidates looking for employment—a ratio of 4 available jobs per candidate. The ratio of available physician positions to physician candidates was 7 to 1—meaning that every physician graduating from a school of public health could have his or her pick of public health jobs and that most would perforce go to doctors without any specialized public health training.[22] The Committee on Professional Education also made great efforts to recruit candidates into public health, conducting 376 office interviews in the course of the year. With funds from the Children's Bureau, the Public Health Service, and the National Foundation for Infantile Paralysis, they set up a "Merit System Unit" to prepare "modern, objective types of examinations" as a way of assisting health and personnel officers identify qualified candidates for their openings.

A survey of schools of public health in 1950 found them overcrowded and underfunded, lacking key faculty members, lacking classroom and laboratory space, and lacking necessary equipment.[23] All were suffering from high levels of financial stress. The schools were under pressure to provide more practical training but the Deans argued that they needed a 70 percent increase in full-time faculty to expand the "applied" fields of instruction. They also stated that they could double the number of students enrolled if they had the necessary financial support for staff, basic operating funds, and construction. The applied fields most frequently in demand were public health administration, environmental sanitation, maternal and child hygiene, industrial hygiene, mental health, medical care organization, public health economics, public health nursing, and health education.[24]

Given this context, it seems hardly surprising that the criteria for accreditation of schools of public health as implemented at mid-century seem undemanding by current standards. The physical facilities required, for

---

[22] Shepard, "Professionalization," p. 148.

[23] Leonard S Rosenfeld, Marjorie Gooch, and Oscar H Levine. *Report on Schools of Public Health in the United States Based on a Survey of Schools of Public Health in 1950.* Public Health Service, U.S. Department of Health Education and Welfare, pub. No. 276. United States Government Printing Office, Washington, DC, 1953.

[24] *Ibid.,* pp. 86–87.

example, were defined (in their entirety) as "lecture rooms, seminar rooms, and adequate laboratory facilities for the teaching of subjects in the field of microbiology, including microscope, culture media, apparatus, etc.; for the teaching of vital statistics, including calculating machines for student use, and apparatus for chart-making, with tabulating machinery available for demonstration purposes and for the teaching of sanitary engineering, including laboratory facilities for the examination of water and sewage and for the demonstration of the basic principles of hydraulics."[25]

For accreditation, the faculty of a school of public health had to consist of at least eight full-time professors. The school had to have "practical autonomy" such that the public health faculty effectively controlled all degree requirements. The most frequently listed fields of faculty of schools of public health in 1953 were, in order, public health practice, microbiology, epidemiology, sanitation, physiological hygiene, vital statistics, biochemistry or nutrition, industrial hygiene, parasitology, public health nursing, health education, maternal and child health, social and economic problems, and mental hygiene. Between 1947 and 1953, the average number of faculty in accredited schools of public health grew from 13 to 19—an increase of 50 percent. The mean ratio of students per faculty member was 4.5, a ratio that was justified by the need for many diverse disciplines and the "intimate personal contact between teacher and pupil in seminars and in field work."[26] Every accredited school was required to have a library consisting of at least 3,000 volumes in the fields of public health and 50 current periodicals.

Perhaps the most interesting part of the accreditation of schools of public health was the evaluation of practical training and fieldwork. Schools had to be located close to local public health services that could be used for "observation and criticism" and these public health services had to be of sufficiently high quality "to make such observation fruitful."[27] Indeed, all the accredited schools reported some sort of functional association with county or city health departments. The Columbia school, for example, shared a building with one of New York City's District Health Centers; the school selected the District Health Officer from a list, provided by the Department of Health, of those eligible for appointment. Johns Hopkins had the Eastern Health District, which was jointly operated by the City Health Department and the school. The School of Public Hygiene, thanks to funds provided by the Rockefeller Foundation, paid the salaries of the District Health Officer and several staff members.

---

[25] Charles-Edward A. Winslow, *The Accreditation of North American Schools of Public Health.* New York: American Public Health Association, 1953, p. 4.

[26] *Ibid.*, p. 11.

[27] *Ibid.*, p. 5.

In Michigan, teams of public health students were sent out to the surrounding county health departments. Each team member spent time working with their corresponding county health worker, handling mail and telephone calls, and getting the "feel" of the work in progress. Later, the students received weekly reports from the corresponding member of the county staff and held regular meetings to discuss the progress of the county's health program. The Kellogg Foundation supported this program by paying 10 percent of the county health department's entire budget. North Carolina's Department of Field Training worked with local health departments in training, consultation, and the provision of educational materials. The recently formed school at Pittsburgh worked with the Pittsburgh Health Department in organizing the work of the Arsenal Health Center, along the lines of the Eastern Health District of Baltimore. Similarly, the Harvard school used its field training program in the Whittier Street Health Unit of the Boston Health Department to train public health, medical, nursing, and social science students. Toronto had its field training in the East York-Leaside Health Unit, with a population of 60,000. The Toronto school of public health paid the salary of the health officer and contributed directly to the budget of the unit. The Department of Public Health at Yale provided surveys of town and city health programs in Connecticut at the request of local health departments. Each year, the students and faculty completed one such survey and presented their results to the local authorities.

In 1951–52, the schools of public health collectively registered 950 students, of whom over 500 were candidates for the M.P.H., 100 for M.S. or M.A., and 100 for the M.S. in Hospital Administration. With the G.I. Bill, the numbers of physicians training in schools of public health had risen sharply for a few years immediately after the war but then began to fall again in 1949.[28] In their place, the schools were admitting increasing numbers of engineers, nurses, and health educators and other students qualified by a bachelor's degree plus experience in public health. Furthermore, 40 percent of all M.P.H. students were from foreign counties and only 16 percent of the United States students were "new recruits" to public health.

Many of the schools offered a vast array of courses: Columbia, for example, offered 127 courses and Michigan almost matched this record with 120 courses. In general, the schools seemed to offer almost as many courses as they had students. The main areas of the curriculum were public health practice, sanitation, vital statistics, and epidemiology, stan-

---

[28] "Public Health Degrees and Certificates Granted in the United States and Canada during the Academic Year, 1949–50," *American Journal of Public Health,* 41, 1951, pp. 217–220.

dard offerings in all the schools; most also offered environmental fields and microbiology.

In the immediate post-war period, many of the schools of public health were involved in curricular reviews and imaginative planning of core courses. For a few years, the concepts of social medicine, social epidemiology, and the ecology of health generated considerable interest. Iago Galdston, Secretary of the New York Academy of Medicine, organized a conference on social medicine in 1947, later publishing the papers as *Social Medicine: Its Derivations and Objectives.*[29] The conferees examined some of the ideas of John Ryle, the first professor of social medicine at Oxford University, and added their own thoughts about the "ecology of health" and the "epidemiology of health." The general concept was that although bacteriology was adequate for understanding many of the infectious diseases, study of the chronic diseases required an understanding of the relationship of health to the physical, social, and economic environment.

These radical ideas prompted faculty in schools of public health to develop new core courses that emphasized the social and economic context of health problems. From now on, they said, the technical skills of bacteriological and epidemiological analysis would have to be embedded within a larger vision of public health. They criticized pre-war curricula as being too narrowly focused on laboratory studies of disease organisms, too little on the social environment. At Harvard, for example, the epidemiologist John E. Gordon declared that "most important of all is to incorporate within the general fabric of public health a more adequate emphasis on social and economic factors. . . ."[30] Harvard instituted two core courses, one on "Human Ecology" and the other on "Community Organization," designed to "orient the public health program to the framework of modern society" by discussing such matters as "the problem of food supply in relation to world population" and "the influences of industry and transportation on human health."[31] The department of public health administration also offered a series of lectures and seminars on "the history of the public health movement" and "the cultural, social, and economic forces bearing on the evolution of the science of public health."[32] Similarly, Columbia reorganized its curriculum around a single required course covering such topics as "the community and its needs," "the evaluation of health status," "the factors which influence the causation and control of disease," and "public health as a community service." At Pitts-

---

[29] Iago Galdston, ed., *Social Medicine: Its Derivations and Objectives.* New York: The Commonwealth Fund, 1949.

[30] As cited in Winslow, *Accreditation*, p. 26.

[31] As cited in Winslow, *Accreditation*, p. 28.

[32] Curran, *Founders of the Harvard School of Public Health*, p. 219.

burgh, Thomas Parran had decided that the curriculum should be organized around "the systematic presentation of illustrative topics which
deal with the interrelation of man and his total environment and with the
political, economic, and social framework within which the health officer
must work."[33] Yale's core course on "Principles and Practice of Public
Health" was similarly organized around a series of interdisciplinary seminars running throughout the academic year. Winslow commented approvingly that the 11 schools of public health constituted "eleven experimental laboratories in which new pedagogic approaches are constantly
being devised."[34]

The overall impression of the accredited schools of public health in
1950 was that they were doing a good job of preparing public health
practitioners through courses and fieldwork, that the numbers of faculty
and students were growing, and that curricular and research innovations
seemed promising. The main complaints of the schools seemed to be lack
of funding to pay faculty, expand space, and purchase equipment. One
other problem, now as earlier, was the fact that the schools of public
health attracted few physicians.[35] Instead, the schools were accepting an
ever-higher proportion of students without health professional training.
Winslow and others made a virtue of necessity, arguing that the many
different types of students gave public health its unique character:

> . . . *public health is not a branch of medicine or of engineering, but a profession
> dedicated to community service which involves the cooperative effort of a dozen
> different disciplines. The fact that doctors and dentists and nurses and engi-
> neers and health educators and microbiologists and statisticians and nutrition-
> ists sit together in our schools and take the same degrees is of incalculable
> importance. It is based on bold assumptions; but it has worked. It provides the
> only sure basis for true cooperative community service in the future. It consti-
> tutes one of the most significant contributions of the United States to the basic
> philosophy of public health.*[36]

---

[33] As cited in Zaga M. Blockstein, *Graduate School of Public Health, University of Pittsburgh,
1948–1974*. Pittsburgh: University of Pittsburgh, 1977, p. 55.

[34] Winslow, *Accreditation*, p. 29.

[35] Henry Vaughan, Dean of the University of Michigan School of Public Health, commented in 1951 that "the physician . . . unfortunately is fast disappearing from the public
health arena, probably for economic reasons," and advocated that the administrative work
of health departments should be taken over by non-medical administrators as most physicians disliked the details of administrative jobs: budget preparation, personnel management, health education, and the like. Henry F. Vaughan, "The Role of the School of Public
Health in Meeting the Man Power Crisis," *American Journal of Public Health*, 41, 1951, 1497–
1502.

[36] Winslow, *Accreditation*, p. 44.

BIOMEDICAL FUNDING IN THE POST-WAR ERA

The war had demonstrated the success of an organized federal effort in financing scientific research; the wartime Committee on Medical Research could point to many successes: the development of atabrine, an effective new treatment for malaria, the therapeutic use of blood derivatives such as gamma globulin, and most notably, the production of huge stocks of the "miracle drug," penicillin. After the war, responsibility for the wartime projects still underway was transferred to the Public Health Service and the National Institute of Health (which became the National Institutes of Health in 1948). In the post-war period, the budget of the National Institutes of Health grew from $180,000 in 1945, to $4 million in 1947, to $46.3 million in 1950, to $81 million in 1955, to $400 million in 1960. The budget continued to grow dramatically, especially under the influence of Mary Lasker and Florence Mahoney as wealthy and persuasive lobbyists, and James Shannon, the forceful and impressive Director of NIH between 1955 and 1968.

In 1944, Thomas Parran, the Surgeon General, had drawn up a grand 10-year plan for his agency, the Public Health Service. Parran envisioned a remarkably complete health service, including public health and medical care, as well as health professional education and medical research:

> *When peace returns, this country should so reorganize and develop its health resource that there will be available to everyone in the population all health and medical services necessary for the preservation and promotion of health, the prevention of disease, and the treatment of illness . . . . It is believed that the use of public funds is fully justified in developing the physical plant for health, in training professional personnel, in supporting both public and private medical and scientific research of broad public interest, and in reducing the individual financial burden resulting from catastrophic illness or chronic disability.*
>
> *The principle is accepted that no one in the United States should be denied access to health and medical services because of economic status, race, geophysical location, or any other non-health factor or condition. It is a duty of governments—local, State, or Federal—to guarantee healthful living conditions and to enable every person to secure freedom from preventable disease.*[37]

Only part of this grand vision was to be realized. Because of the hostility and deep pockets of the American Medical Association and their allies, neither the comprehensive expansion of the public health service nor the institution of national health insurance would prove politically

---

[37] Thomas Parran, "Proposed Ten-year Postwar Program. The United States Public Health Service," November 1, 1944. Parran Papers, Modern Manuscripts, History of Medicine Division, National Library of Medicine.

possible. Thomas Parran himself was relieved of his position as Surgeon General and replaced by the more malleable Leonard Scheele. There was no lack of money to spend. In 1946, the Hospital Survey and Construction Act, or Hill-Burton program, was passed to finance the construction of community hospitals, initially providing $75 million a year for five years, and eventually pouring $3.7 billion into new hospital construction. The Hill-Burton program was strongly supported by the American Hospital Association and the American Medical Association; it provided new facilities for medical practice without threatening in any way the method of paying for health services. Indeed, Hill-Burton had a specific provision prohibiting federal involvement in setting hospital policy.[38] The system of Veterans Administration hospitals was also greatly expanded and tied in more closely to local medical schools.

Scheele had earlier been associate director of the National Cancer Institute and was now, as Surgeon General, responsible for the National Institutes of Health. Like hospital construction, medical research had many friends and seemingly no enemies. Cancer and heart institutes had been the first, mental health and dental institutes followed, and then came a succession of other special institutes targeted toward a specific disease (diabetes, arthritis), body part (eye, kidney), or stage in the life cycle (child health, aging). The institutes grew and grew wealthy; they also gave away most of their funds to universities and medical schools in the form of research grants. Because the medical schools and the American Medical Association had opposed the direct provision of federal funds to medical education—nursing an avid suspicion of any form of governmental intervention or control—the NIH research grants proved a politically acceptable way of funneling money to the medical schools. No federal bureaucrats were deciding the dollar amounts given to a particular school: grants were awarded on the decisions of peer review committees composed of non-federal experts in the particular field of research. Liberals, conservatives, medical school deans, and researchers were all happy with the system, and members of Congress were pleased to bankroll such a popular and uncontroversial program.[39]

Schools of public health would have had no objection whatsoever to direct federal funding—assuming only that it were relatively generous. But public health schools were generally lumped in with medical schools

[38] Paul Starr, *The Social Transformation of American Medicine*. New York: Basic Books, p.p. 348–351.

[39] Stephen P. Strickland, *Politics, Science, and Dread Disease: A Short History of United States Medical Research Policy*. Cambridge, MA: Harvard University Press, 1972. See also Eli Ginzberg and Anna B. Dutka, *The Financing of Biomedical Research*. Baltimore: The Johns Hopkins University Press, 1989.

(and later with health professional education) when it came to setting federal policy, so they had to compete with medical schools for research grants—in a grant system dominated by powerful medical school professors. The historic funders of schools of public health, the great foundations, were well aware of the increasingly important role of the federal government in financing medical research and education. Some of their officers were perhaps disappointed with the achievements of the early schools of public health, especially in their failure to spread the preventive point of view throughout medical education; in any case, they now directed their interest toward building departments of preventive medicine and community medicine within medical schools. The Pan American Health Organization, which had sent so many Latin American students to North American schools during the war years, now came to believe that training in the United States was not very relevant to the problems of developing countries, and argued that international students were best trained in countries with similar health problems, culture, and climate.[40]

Adding to the woes of schools of public health was the period of deepening conservatism from about 1948 through the late 1950s. The mood in government and on campuses changed in the atmosphere of the Cold War. McCarthyism associated any advocacy of public health agendas or national health insurance with "socialized medicine" and identified this in turn with socialism or Communism. When Thomas Parran, who had been ousted as Surgeon General, took over as Dean of the new Pittsburgh School of Public Health, he was attacked as a "Communist," who favored socialized medicine and compulsory health insurance.[41] (The Mellon Trustees who had financed the school poured over Parran's past speeches and publications and decided that the charges were unfounded.) In the late 1940s and early 1950s, many of the most articulate and outspoken public health leaders were under attack, silenced, or were losing their positions and their influence.

A DEEPENING CRISIS: PUBLIC HEALTH SCHOOLS AND DEPARTMENTS IN THE 1950S

In the early 1950s, schools of public health were attempting both to maintain educational standards and to admit increasing numbers of students, in spite of the fact that most students were unable to finance

---

[40] Marcos Charnes, "Problems Confronting Foreign Students Beginning Professional Education in the United States and in Adapting it to Practice at Home," in *The Professional Education of Students from Other Lands*, ed., Irwin T. Sanders, New York: Council on Social Work Education, 1962.

[41] *Ibid.*, p.63.

their own education, state governments only reluctantly provided minimal funding, the foundations had lost much of their enthusiasm for
financing public health education, and international agencies were ques-
tioning the value of American schools for their international students.
Schools of public health were all complaining that they lacked sufficient
funds for operating expenses and faculty salaries. We need to understand the suffering of the schools in the context of the growing conservatism of the country during the early years of the Cold War, growing
popular suspicion of government programs, and seething hostility to
even such cost-effective public health measures as the fluoridation of
water supplies. We also need to see the schools of public health in the
context of a massive expansion in funding for biomedical research as an
uncontroversial way to pour money into the health enterprise in the
post-war era.

It is hardly surprising that the schools of public health all settled on
essentially the same survival strategy, which they pursued with greater
or lesser enthusiasm, and with greater or lesser reluctance, depending on
the orientation and interests of their faculty and deans. They would apply
for research grants and use the research funds to pay the salaries of additional faculty members, on the grounds that new faculty could spend
some of their time teaching and some of their time on funded research. In
1950, on an average across schools of public health, faculty spent 40 percent time on teaching, 40 percent on research, 10 percent on administration and 10 percent on service. Averages, however, are misleading because they mask the wide variation between schools of public health and
even between different departments within a particular school. What hap-
pened was that, if the faculty of a particular department was devoted
mainly to teaching or to "service" (public health practice), the numbers of
faculty stayed stable or gradually declined. If the department was devoted to research, and was reasonably successful at funding that research,
the department grew, added more people, consumed more space and
equipment, published a steady stream of research papers and reports,
and generally gave the impression of being a dynamic and productive
place. Size begat size, growth begat growth, and research success bred
research success. Over time, the results could be dramatic, with some
schools and departments growing at an impressive rate and others ap-
pearing moribund. A few schools, especially Hopkins and Harvard, grew
large and prosperous. Between them, Hopkins and Harvard had 40 percent of all faculty involved in research, trained most of the faculty for
smaller schools, and generally dominated the field. Smaller or less prosperous schools did their best to emulate the research ideal, to garner their
own grant funds, and to grow their own faculty.

Robert Korstad, in his history of the North Carolina School of Public
Health, has effectively shown how this dynamic played out in the devel-

opment of that school.[42] In 1935, the school began as a Division of Public Health in the Medical School, using the new federal funding provided by the Social Security Act; in 1940, it became an independent school of public health, with the eminent Milton Rosenau as its first Director. The school received a small appropriation from the university, some funds from the Public Health Service, and tuition from students. Rosenau recruited part-time faculty from the State Board of Health, obtained part-time teaching assistance from various members of the medical school faculty, and himself taught epidemiology. The Public Health Service supported two faculty members: a professor of public health administration and a professor of sanitary engineering. At first, the school offered a three-month course for public health officers, then developed programs in venereal disease control, public health nursing, and health education—all practice-oriented subjects. The school offered short training courses for armed services personnel and also took in foreign students during the war.

After the war, Edward McGavran, described as a "dyed-in-the-wool field man," became Dean of the school. The Kellogg Foundation supported a large field training program, including short courses, in-service training, supervised field experiences, apprenticeship training, and residencies. McGavran was an enthusiast for public health practice but struggled with the North Carolina state legislature, which resisted expenditures on the grounds that it wished only to support students from North Carolina, whereas the school was admitting students from all over the South, and many international students as well. Meanwhile, the legislature appropriated funds that, combined with federal support under the Hill-Burton program, were sufficient to build a hospital and expand the medical school. The University also built schools of nursing and dentistry. But while buildings were going up all over campus, the school of public health lacked classroom and laboratory space. McGavran lacked operating funds, teaching staff and teaching assistants, administrative staff, and the ability to give raises and replace key personnel. The school of public health paid salaries well below those of the other schools on campus and below the "market value" of persons qualified to fill the positions. Furthermore, the University refused to maintain the field training programs, which were admittedly expensive undertakings in terms of staff time and travel.

McGavran was a determined public health advocate who defined public health as "the scientific diagnosis and treatment of the body politic."[43] He believed that public health practitioners should be able to pro-

---

[42] Robert R. Korstad, *Dreaming of a Time: The School of Public Health, The University of North Carolina at Chapel Hill, 1939-1989*. School of Public Health, University of North Carolina at Chapel Hill, 1990.

[43] Edward G. McGavran, "What Is Public Health?" *Canadian Journal of Public Health*, 44 1953:441–51.

vide analyses of the economy, the political power structure of the community, and the forces determining the acceptance or rejection of progressive change and development. He faced an uphill battle: the Korean War and the increasingly conservative texture of the times favored narrow scientific solutions to health problems rather than a broad social and political understanding of public health. By the mid-fifties, Korstad delicately notes, there was "a perceptible tension between solidarity and individualism" in the school of public health.[44] The Public Health Service and the National Institutes of Health provided categorical grant funding to selected faculty but very little funding for core public health activities.

McGavran tried to hold the faculty together but found it was an impossible task, with the growing pressures for individual entrepreneurial activity, the increasingly uneven development of departments, and the rewards available to those who were successful in obtaining external funding.[45] The department of biostatistics, successful in obtaining research and teaching funds, grew dramatically. So did parasitology and experimental medicine (later renamed environmental sciences and engineering), although McGavran complained that the latter was really an "institute of research" entirely separate from the real work of a school of public health. Epidemiology also thrived under the leadership of John Cassel. But other departments fared poorly: mental health had only one faculty member for several years and, when that individual left, had no faculty at all. The large field training program, which in the early 1950s had engaged the total faculty and all of the students for one day a week at four field centers within a 50 mile radius of the school, was eliminated. The enterprise had been exhilarating, time-consuming, and expensive. "But it was a superb experiment" said McGavran, "and for two brief years the School of Public Health demonstrated to students, practitioners, and ourselves that there was a public health team."[46]

Thus, even a Director who strongly favored field training and distrusted departments devoted to research was unable to resist the pressures favoring research over practical training. The North Carolina school did receive money from the Hill-Rhodes training funds at the end of the 1950s, and the 1960s ushered in an era of growth with increasing research funds and increasing faculty salaries. Successful department chairs built up their faculty by bringing in faculty members on grant (soft) money and then trying to get them hired on state (hard) money. There were battles over space—the people getting research grants constantly needed more space, more laboratories, more offices, and were taking them away from the departments that were slow-growing or static. In the 1960s, many of

---

[44] Korstad, *Dreaming of a Time*, p. 84.
[45] *Ibid.*, p. 86.
[46] *Ibid.*, p. 89.

the non-research faculty, such as the women who had led the public health education department through the 1950s, simply left.

A later self-study of the North Carolina school pointedly noted that relationships with local communities and the state had deteriorated "as departments were concerned with the federal dollar and were worshiping the idols in Washington and Bethesda."[47] Many faculty members felt no particular obligation to health agencies at the state or county level as shown by their complete lack of interest in the activities of the North Carolina Public Health Association. Faculty members whose careers centered on research were reluctant to spend time training local health workers. In return, the state legislature offered the school little support. As a result of these dynamics, all the service-oriented departments that had failed to grow in over a decade of federal support—the departments of health administration, health education, maternal and child health, mental health, public health nursing, and public health nutrition—were bundled into a single department of community health practice and administration.

The same dynamics were at work in other schools of public health. The available funding—and the faculty members who were suited by education, experience, and personality to succeed in the research system—shaped the institutions and drove their priorities. At Johns Hopkins in the late 1940s and early 1950s, the epidemiology department was completely dominated by laboratory-focused polio research generously funded by the Foundation for Infantile Paralysis. The work of David Bodian and others at the Hopkins school certainly played an essential role in laying the scientific basis for a successful polio vaccine; the point here is that other unfunded, or underfunded, activities were allowed to slide. Thus the Eastern Health District, which had been the pride and joy of the epidemiology department in the 1930s, expired quietly in the early 1950s. According to a survey of recent M.P.H. graduates in 1955, the increased emphasis on research was also hurting the quality of teaching. A subcommittee of the admissions committee, concerned that M.P.H. applications were falling, reported back: "The complaint was made that the staff was more concerned with research and affairs outside the school than with teaching, that lectures were hastily prepared and frequently dull."[48]

In this environment, graduate students who helped the professor with his research were of more interest than M.P.H. students, who merely absorbed rather than produced research results. At Hopkins, Elmer McCollum, the professor of chemical hygiene (later biochemistry)

---

[47] *Ibid.*, p. 136.
[48] "Report of Sub-Committee of Applications and Curriculum Committee on Alumni and their MPH Curriculum Suggestions," 1955, p. 10. The Johns Hopkins University Archives. President's Papers, School of Hygiene, 745.

had started the practice of insisting that all his students must work on some aspect of his nutrition studies. These all involved feeding experimental rats different combinations of carefully prepared foodstuffs—adding or eliminating one specific substance at a time—and then measuring the effects of each diet on the weight and health of the rats. The labor force of students who participated in the rat nutrition studies produced a vast number of research papers, most of them co-authored with the professor. This industrial mode of research organization was easily adaptable to other forms of laboratory research and, in time, to other quantitative public health disciplines.

The system of research funding, however, did not work well for field research, public health practice, public health administration, the social sciences, history, politics, law, anthropology, or (at least at this juncture) economics. So within the schools of public health in the 1950s, the laboratory sciences tended to thrive, whereas public health practice and other non-quantitative disciplines suffered. Intellectually, and in the curriculum, there was a state of uneven development. The community-based orientation of the 1930s had disappeared and the field training programs all essentially collapsed.

The Hopkins M.P.H. students who had been queried in 1955 had asked for more instruction in the history, theory, principles, and philosophy of public health.[49] They complained of the required microbiology course: "the laboratory work was too detailed, too mechanical and too unproductive in developing the student's thinking."[50] One student suggested "the general principles of public health administration, field studies in public health, and social medicine and medical care be combined in one comprehensive required course, using the Eastern Health District and the Medical Care Clinic of the Hospital as a joint administrative practice unit for this purpose."[51] In general, the Hopkins students and alumni asked for more attention to problems of chronic diseases, mental illness, and medical care organization; they expressed a desire for a better understanding of social and economic issues, and they wanted a clear overall vision or philosophy of public health.

By the mid 1950s, schools of public health were being pulled in different directions. Much of the rhetoric of change suggested that, as the biological sciences had been needed to solve the problems of infectious disease, so the social sciences were needed to solve the problems of the chronic diseases. Thus the Dean of the Hopkins school, Ernest L. Stebbins, urged the faculty of schools of public health not to shut themselves up in their laboratories but to be actively involved in service to their local com-

[49] *Ibid.*, p. 9.
[50] *Ibid.*, p. 13.
[51] *Ibid*, as cited, p. 15.

munity. "Knowledge of the natural history, the basic etiology, and means of prevention of heart disease," he contended, "may come from sociologic studies rather than from the biological laboratory."[52] A committee of the faculty, popularly termed the "Crystal Ball Committee," suggested new areas of research more relevant to the major health problems of the day: epidemiological and field studies of cancer and chronic diseases, epidemiological studies of mental illness, research into the social determinants of illness, child development studies, health promotion methods, medical care organization, accident prevention, and research on radiation hazards.[53] But the Committee also stated that they did not favor "a marked expansion of the school activities into these areas if it means that the basic science program would undergo a fundamental change."[54] In other words, they knew what the problems were and what new types of research should be done but they also didn't want to change.

As the Hopkins faculty struggled with their crystal ball, the financial situation of the school was worsening. A new Development Committee, chaired by environmental engineer Abel Wolman, spent two years studying the problem and then concluded that the school should abandon its M.P.H. program entirely. Instead, Hopkins would focus on its doctoral programs leading to the Dr.P.H. and the Sc.D. or Ph.D. degree.[55] Doctoral students were research students; their education did not take away from the research program, but fueled it. Admission to the Doctor of Public Health degree would be restricted to those who already held a doctoral degree in the medical, biological, or health sciences. Only a few students who found it impossible to remain at the school long enough to complete their doctorate would be allowed to terminate their academic work with an M.P.H. degree. Describing this as a program of "advanced post-graduate education," the Development Committee report explained: "Admittedly, the admission policy is designed to eliminate students who either have not had medical training or who are strongly deficient in the biological or health sciences."[56] Such students could and should be trained at "other institutions."

---

[52] Ernest L. Stebbins, "Contributions of the Graduate School of Public Health—Past, Present, and Future," *American Journal of Public Health*, 47, 1957, 1508–1512.

[53] Roger M. Herriott, "Report to the Applications and Curriculum Committee by the 'Crystal Ball' Committee Appointed to Consider 'Where the Field of Public Health is Going'," May 16, 1955. Alan Mason Chesney Archives of the Johns Hopkins Medical Institutions, Crystal Ball Committee, Box 22 Hygiene.

[54] *Ibid.*, p. 11.

[55] Abel Wolman, "A Revision of the Educational Program in the Johns Hopkins University School of Hygiene and Public Health," March 1958. The Rockefeller Foundation Archives, Tarrytown, New York.

[56] *Ibid.*, p. 4.

As the Hopkins faculty—against the advice of their own Dean—withdrew into their laboratories, they further distanced themselves from the problems of local health departments. And the health departments were in a sorry state. In the 1950s, federal grants-in-aid to the states for public health programs steadily declined with the total dollar amounts falling from $45 million in 1950 to $33 million in 1959. Given inflation, this represented a dramatic decline in purchasing power.[57] Public health departments were caught in a downward spiral. Lacking funds, they couldn't bring in new people or begin new programs; lack of new people and programs gave them an aura of failure and irrelevance. Health departments ran underfunded programs with underqualified people who answered to unresponsive bureaucrats. When state legislators wanted to start new programs, they tended to overlook the dull and unimaginative state health departments, regarded as backwaters for those who could not succeed in the private sector. Public health officials were expressing "frustrations, disappointments, dissatisfactions, and discontentments" said John W. Knutson in his Presidential Address to the American Public Health Association in 1957.[58] As Jesse Aronson, director of local health services in New Jersey, explained:

> *The full-time health officer is frequently, because of inadequate budget and staff, limited in his activities to a series of routine clinical responsibilities in a child health station, a tuberculosis clinic, a venereal disease clinic, an immunization session, and communicable disease diagnosis and treatment. He has little or no time for community health education, the study of health problems and trends, the initiation of newer programs in diabetes control, cancer control, rheumatic fever prophylaxis, nutrition education, and radiation control. In a great many areas the health officer position has been vacant year after year with little real hope of filling it. In these situations, even the pretense of public health leadership is left behind and local medical practitioners provide these services on an hourly basis.[59]*

Between 1947 and 1957, the numbers of students being trained in schools of public health fell by half. Alarmed, Ernest Stebbins of Johns Hopkins and Hugh Leavell of Harvard, representing the Association of Schools of Public Health, walked the halls of the United States Congress

---

[57] Milton Terris, "The Changing Face of Public Health," *American Journal of Public Health,* 49, 1959, p. 1119.

[58] John W. Knutson, "Ferment in Public Health," *American Journal of Public Health,* 47, 1957, 1489. See also the generally depressing statements by Leonard Woodcock, Hugh R. Leavell, "Where Are We Going in Public Health?" *American Journal of Public Health,* 46, 1956, 278–82.

[59] Jesse B. Aronson, "The Politics of Public Health—Reactions and Summary," *American Journal of Public Health,* 49, 1959, p. 311.

to urge its members to support public health education. They found an especially sympathetic audience in Senator Lister Hill and Representative George M. Rhodes, and in 1958, Congress enacted a two-year emergency program authorizing $1 million a year in federal grants to be divided among the accredited schools of public health.

The First National Conference on Public Health Training in 1958 noted that these funds had provided 1,000 traineeships and had greatly improved morale in public health agencies. The Conference further requested appropriations for teaching grants and construction costs for teaching facilities, and urged that faculty salary support be provided for teaching. Their report concluded with a stirring appeal to value public health education as vital to national defense:

> *The great crises of the future may not come from a foreign enemy…"D" day for disease and death is everyday. The battle line is in our own community. To hold that battle line we must daily depend on specially trained physicians, nurses, biochemists, public health engineers, and other specialists properly organized for the normal protection of the homes, the schools, and the work places of some unidentified city somewhere in America. That city has, today, neither the personnel nor the resources of knowledge necessary to protect it.[60]*

President Eisenhower signed the Hill-Rhodes bill, authorizing $1 million annually in formula grants for accredited schools of public health and $2 million annually for five years for project training grants; between 1957 and 1963 the United States Congress would appropriate $15 million to support public health trainees. The worst of the crisis was over. In the 1960s, Lister Hill would continue to champion the cause of the schools of public health in the Senate and John E. Fogarty became their main supporter in the House. The Congress raised the ceiling on the formula grants, provided grants-in-aid for training to state health departments, and authorized special training grants, fellowships for faculty development, and construction grants for schools of public health.

New Life in the Sixties

The federal government now began to reverse the damage that had been done to public health by providing traineeships, formula grants, and project grants to develop new curricular areas. The downward trend in public health enrollments was halted; in 1960, student enrollments again began to climb. The Association of Schools of Public Health happily dis-

---

[60] Report of the National Conference on Public Health Training to the Surgeon General of the Public Health Service, July 28–30, 1958. Washington, DC: United States Department of Health, Education, and Welfare, p. 3.

TABLE D-1   Federal Support for Schools of Public Health[1]

Year	Traineeships	Project Grants	Formula Grants
1957	1,000,000		
1960	2,000,000		1,000,000
1963	4,000,000	2,000,000	1,900,000
1966	7,000,000	4,000,000	3,500,000
1969	8,000,000	4,917,000	4,554,000
1972	8,400,000	4,517,000	5,554,000

[1]Table from *Higher Education for Public Health*, p. 164.

cussed the "ferment" in schools of public health around the new, or newly recognized, problems of chronic illness, mental disorder, air pollution, medical care organization, aging, injuries, and radiation hazards. The new federal funds provided some basic operating costs but also encouragement to explore targeted areas of research and training. New schools of public health were created at the University of California, Los Angeles, and in Puerto Rico, and many schools expanded their previously cramped facilities. In 1963, the federal government doubled the ceiling on formula grants and also began offering construction grants to schools of public health.

This was an exciting time for the schools; between 1960 and 1964, the total number of applicants to schools of public health more than doubled; the number of faculty members increased by 50 percent; the average space occupied increased by 50 percent; and the average income of the schools more than doubled.[61] New faculty appointments were made in such fields as medical care organization, social and behavioral sciences, public health administration, human ecology, radiation sciences, population studies, and international health.

The newly created Agency for International Development (AID) encouraged schools of public health to develop international health training programs whose students would become "ambassadors of American science" abroad.[62] By 1965, the whole country seemed to have become concerned about the "population explosion," and the United States Congress was voting money to provide technical assistance, often in the form of contraceptives, to the developing world.

The passage of Medicare and Medicaid legislation in 1965 generated

---

[61] Elizabeth Fee and Barbara Rosenkrantz, "Professional Education for Public Health in the United States," in Elizabeth Fee and Roy M. Acheson, eds. *A History of Education in Public Health: Health that Mocks the Doctors' Rules*. Oxford: Oxford University Press; 1991, 230–271.

[62] Minutes, April 7–8, 1964, Executive Session, Association of Schools of Public Health, pp. 6–7. Alan Mason Chesney Archives of the Johns Hopkins Medical Institutions, RG 1, Box 48.

considerable excitement in schools of public health. State health agencies were concerned about being able to monitor and evaluate medical care services and wanted the schools of public health to provide the scientific basis for rational decision-making in health services delivery. They also wanted the schools to provide training for medical care administrators and financial managers. In 1966, a Special Study Commission of the Association of Schools of Public Health estimated that 6,220 new positions in medical care administration required graduate-level educational preparation.[63] The United States Public Health Service curtailed its usual grant application procedures to provide quick funding to schools of public health willing to provide short courses in health services administration. As in the 1930s, short courses would be developed to meet the urgency of the national need.

In the context of the Civil Rights movement and the demand for more community participation in health care, education, and other sectors of civil life, the Kennedy administration supported the movement away from mental hospitals and toward community mental health centers, run on an outpatient basis. Community mental health centers were financed by the federal government and locally controlled, thus largely bypassing the states. Many of the other programs of the 1960s and 1970s would be created as independent ventures, thus directly or indirectly weakening the role of the states and of state health departments. In the year before he died, Kennedy began developing an anti-poverty program and, after his assassination, President Johnson expanded this into the "War on Poverty."[64] As part of this general effort, the Office of Equal Opportunity (OEO) helped to start 100 neighborhood health centers and the Department of Health, Education, and Welfare (HEW) supported another 50.[65] The aim of these health centers was to provide comprehensive primary care services and to encourage community participation in running the organizations. The centers were, however, dependent on public funds for their survival, and an ambitious plan to build 1,000 centers across the country was never realized.

In the generally progressive social ferment of the 1960s, a strong environmental movement developed around the catalyst provided by publication of Rachel Carson's *Silent Spring* in 1962.[66] Earth Day in 1970 at-

---

[63] Report of the Special Study Committee, "The Role of Schools of Public Health in Relation to Trends in Medical Care Programs in the United States and Canada," April 6, 1966. Association of Schools of Public Health, Alan Mason Chesney Archives of the Johns Hopkins Medical Institutions, RG 1, Box 48.

[64] Karen Davis and Cathy Schoen, *Health and the War on Poverty*. Washington DC: Brookings Institution, 1978.

[65] Paul Starr, *The Social Transformation of American Medicine*, p. 371.

[66] Rachel Carson, *Silent Spring*. Boston: Houghton Mifflin, 1962.

tracted some 20 million Americans in demonstrations against assaults against nature; by 1990, Earth Day brought out 200 million participants in 140 countries.[67] Within the federal government, the environmental movement spurred the creation of the Environmental Protection Agency (EPA) and passage of the Clean Air Act of 1970. At the same time, labor mobilization and public distress over the toll taken by industrial accidents and mining disasters prompted the creation of the Occupational Health and Safety Administration (OSHA) and the National Institute of Occupational Safety and Health (NIOSH).

Environmental protection agencies, like the neighborhood health centers and the community mental health centers, were organizationally independent of state health departments, although they were clearly important agencies for the public's health. Questions of the definition of public health now became more problematic: public health in the broad sense included many of the activities and responsibilities of a wide variety of agencies: the work of departments of public health now represented only one aspect of public health: public health as narrowly defined. At the federal level, public health was also losing administrative focus. The formation of the Department of Health, Education, and Welfare in 1953 had reduced the visibility and centrality of the Public Health Service; further reorganizations and changes continued to diminish its role. By 1975, it was clear that the Surgeon General no longer functioned as the head of the Public Health Service. Instead, the Office of the Assistant Secretary of Health had been strengthened and the main health agencies, including the National Institutes of Health, the Food and Drug Administration, and the Center for Disease Control reported directly to him. The Surgeon General had become a figurehead, a spokesperson without direct line authority.

Throughout the 1960s and early 1970s, schools of public health thrived with federal funding available for both teaching programs and research. In 1960, there were 12 accredited schools of public health in the United States; 8 more were added between 1965 and 1975. Between 1965 and 1972, student enrolments again doubled, with the large majority being candidates for the M.P.H. degree. The trend to admit more students who were not physicians, and more students without prior experience in public health, continued. Whereas in 1946–1947, 61 percent of all students admitted to schools of public health for the M.P.H. were physicians, by 1968–1969, physicians constituted only 19 percent of M.P.H. candidates.[68] Many schools admitted students fresh from their undergraduate degrees.

---

[67] J.R. McNeil, *Something New Under the Sun: An Environmental History of the Twentieth-Century World*. New York: W.W. Norton, 2000, p. 339.

[68] T. Hall et al. *Professional Health Manpower for Community Health Programs*. Report Compiled by School of Public Health of the University of North Carolina at Chapel Hill, North Carolina. 1973.

Graduate Programs in Other Schools of the University

Along with the growth in the accredited schools of public health came a rapid growth in other forms of public health and health services education. Some of these were graduate programs in a variety of university departments and in schools of engineering, medical schools, schools of business administration, schools of nursing, schools of social work, and schools of education and communication. They were offering degrees in such fields as environmental health, health management and administration, nutrition, public health nursing, and health education. Somewhat to the distress of accredited schools of public health, most employers did not distinguish between accredited and non-accredited programs.[69] By 1975, there were some 43 graduate programs in health administration offered in schools of public or business administration and 15 graduate programs in nutrition offered by departments of home economics, education, and human development. More than 30 nursing schools offered graduate programs in public health nursing and community nursing. In addition, all nurses enrolled in baccalaureate programs received some public health education; associate degree programs and diploma programs generally did not provide this. About 30 schools of education or allied health offered graduate health education programs and at least 59 technical and engineering schools and departments of environmental sciences offered graduate training in environmental health.

In addition to this flourishing of programs across university campuses, there had been a dramatic growth of junior and community colleges. By the mid 1970s, some 69,000 students were enrolled in various allied health programs.[70] Universities were setting up popular baccalaureate programs in health administration, environmental engineering, health education, and nutrition. Some 58 academic units offered four-year undergraduate programs in environmental engineering; 25 colleges offered undergraduate degrees in community health education, 75 in school health education, and 83 in nutrition.

Schools of public health were, at best, ambivalent about undergraduate education in public health. Several schools of public health (Berkeley, UCLA, North Carolina, Michigan, and Puerto Rico) had earlier offered undergraduate degrees but tended to phase these out in the 1960s; some however were adding new programs in response to perceived manpower needs. As the Milbank Commission Report noted in 1975, public health education was a growth industry with no apparent end in sight. But the system was fractured: although 5,000 graduate degrees in public health were awarded each year, approximately half of higher education for pub-

---

[69] Cecil G. Sheps, *Higher Education for Public Health: A Report of the Milbank Memorial Fund Commission*. New York: Prodist, 1976, p. 82.

[70] *Ibid.*, p. 86.

lic health was occurring outside of accredited schools of public health. Were schools of public health still needed?

THE THREATENED WITHDRAWAL OF FEDERAL FUNDS

Evidently, President Richard Nixon thought not, for in 1973, he recommended terminating federal support for schools of public health and the discontinuation of all research training grants, direct traineeships, and fellowships. This sent shockwaves through a system that had grown dependent on a steady flow of federal funding for its basic support. The strain of the funding cutback threats is reflected in the papers from a Macy Foundation-funded Conference held at the Rockefeller Foundation's Study and Conference Center in Bellagio, Italy, in 1974. In the volume published from that conference, Cecil Sheps, then Vice Chancellor of the University of North Carolina, noted that leading schools of public health were wondering "seriously and agonizingly" about their future.[71] The participants offered a generally gloomy assessment of public health education. According to Russell Nelson of the Johns Hopkins Medical Institutions, corridor talk at his campus said that public health was dead. At Hopkins, moves to absorb the School of Public Health into the medical school had been held back mainly because the medical school faculty were unenthusiastic.[72] Herbert Longnecker, the President of Tulane University, gave voice to his medical school's position when he said, "I think I am correct in stating that the record of fundamental scientific contributions of schools of public health is minor."[73] John C. Hume, now Dean of the Johns Hopkins School of Public Health, spoke about the changes that he had experienced over 20 years as a consequence of the patterns of federal support for biomedical research. The once cohesive nature of the school had been lost, he said: there was little shared conversation, and no coherent teaching program. The autonomy and independence of departments and faculty did encourage initiative but also resulted in isolation and fragmentation. Instead of a unified school of public health, the departments constituted "a series of mini-schools with limited interests." Hume noted that his major problem as Dean was to cope with the fiscal tides—the waxing and waning of federal enthusiasm for particular topics. In the 1960s, for example, population studies had been elevated in impor-

---

[71] Cecil G. Sheps, "Trends in Schools of Public Health in the United States Since World War 11," in *Schools of Public Health: Present and Future, Report of a Macy Conference*, ed., John Z. Bowers and Elizabeth F. Purcell. New York: Josiah Macy, Jr. Foundation, 1974, p. 9.

[72] Russell A. Nelson, "Organizational Relationships of Schools of Public Health with Schools of Medicine," in *Schools of Public Health: Present and Future*, pp. 11–14.

[73] Herbert E. Longnecker, "Organizational Relationships of Schools of Public Health with Universities," in *Schools of Public Health: Present and Future*, pp. 19–24.

tance with the influx of new funding, but by the end of the decade, this interest had largely evaporated.[74]

Representatives of all the schools of public health appeared to agree with J. Thomas Grayson of the University of Washington's relatively new and rapidly-expanding School of Public Health and Community Medicine: "The greatest immediate challenge to the School of Public Health and Community Medicine is the uncertainty of federal funding brought about by the administration's announced intention to end, or greatly curtail, federal support for the training of public health manpower, coupled with a similar proposal to decrease support for research training."[75] The one student representative at the conference, identified as recent graduate Frank C. Ramsey, stated the students' distress with an educational system focused on soft money:

> *The financing of the school I attended is such that the departmental heads and faculty members are mainly responsible for raising money. Most of the funds come from federal sources and virtually all of them go into research. The heads of departments with popular programs find it easier to raise funds than is the case with heads of departments with less research-oriented programs. The grant system influences the school's organization, function, and orientation . . . [it] places constraints on the type of professionals employed and the work performed . . . [among the students] there was a fairly general belief that solutions to societal problems were being sacrificed on the altar of scientific research.[76]*

Some of the threatened funding cuts were restored, but the trend in the 1970s was toward ever more reliance on targeted research funding, thus exacerbating the problems to which Ramsey had referred. In 1976, the Milbank Memorial Fund issued its extensive report, *Higher Education for Public Health.*[77] The Milbank Commission, chaired by Cecil Sheps, asked the usual questions: Why was there not a closer relationship between professional education and professional practice? Should education change or should the practice model? Could departments of community medicine in medical schools serve some of the functions of schools of public health?

---

[74] John C. Hume, "The Future of Schools of Public Health: The Johns Hopkins University School of Hygiene and Public Health," in *Schools of Public Health: Present and Future*, pp 60–69.

[75] J. Thomas Grayston, "New Approaches in Schools of Public Health: The University of Washington School of Public Health and Community Medicine," in *Schools of Public Health: Present and Future* p. 58.

[76] Frank C. Ramsey, "Observations of a Recent Graduate of a School of Public Health," in *Schools of Public Health: Present and Future*, pp. 130–133.

[77] Milbank Memorial Fund, *Higher Education for Public Health: A Report of the Milbank Memorial Fund Commission.* New York: Prodist, 1976,

And, most sharply: Had schools of public health become so dependent on federal funds that "their policies and programs are determined by dollars available and they no longer control their own destiny?"[78]

In place of a public health educational system that Cecil Sheps described as "chaotic, wasteful, and dysfunctional," the Commission proposed what they considered a more rational structure.[79] This sounded rather like an updated version of the original Wickliffe Rose design of 1914. There would be a three-tiered system of public health education. Schools of public health should educate people at the highest level to assume leadership positions; they should train the public health executives who must have a broad knowledge of the entire field and be able to function within the full range of the knowledge base for public health.

Next, programs in graduate schools should prepare the large number of professionals engaged in providing clearly differentiated specialty services, e.g., public health nurses, health educators, and environmental health specialists. Third, although Commission members were uncertain about the value of baccalaureate programs, they might provide some of the "trained entry-level personnel."[80] The Commission defined the "three elements of the knowledge base generic to public health" as:

- Epidemiology and Biostatistics
- Social Policy and the History and Philosophy of Public Health
- Management and Organization for Public Health

Their report also listed a series of "cognate fields": clinical sciences, biomedical sciences, environmental sciences, social sciences, management sciences, law, and ethics that might well be provided by other departments of the university. The schools of public health should focus on the three core curricular areas and should receive basic core support from the federal government for doing so. They should also serve as regional resources by assisting faculties in medical and other health-related schools to develop teaching programs and research in public health. Different schools would serve as national centers of excellence for specific fields but "should avoid setting up special programs in every new area simply because funding is available."[81] Instead, faculty should become involved in the operation of community health services in areas relevant to their areas of academic responsibility, thus offering supervised field experience for aspiring public health practitioners. In general, the Commission proposed that schools of public health become smaller and more focused

---

[78] L.E. Burney, "Foreword," *Higher Education for Public Health*, p. viii.
[79] *Higher Education for Public Health*, p. 211.
[80] *Ibid.*, p. 98.
[81] *Ibid.*, p. 123.

on broad research plans rather than grasping at every funding opportunity. Nor should they do basic laboratory work that could as well be done in a medical school; instead, they should recognize and value their unique interdisciplinary character and craft research plans that drew upon these strengths and were relevant to the regions and communities in which they were located.

The Milbank Commission Report offered faint praise for the system of research driven by changing federal funding priorities: "This is not always bad, as it sometimes results in research that is realistically related to the needs and interests of the nation."[82] By implication, schools would do better if their faculty could design their own research within a broad framework established by the needs of public health in practice. Indeed, Sheps urged faculty to take strong advocacy positions as "academic freedom, like all liberties, is bound to atrophy unless exercised."[83]

The specific recommendations of the Milbank Commission had little impact. No dramatic redesign of public health education could work when the underlying forces driving the system continued unabated. Indeed, under President Ronald Reagan, the pressures intensified. In 1981, his administration consolidated numerous federal health programs into two block grants, cut the total funds by 25 percent, and gave the remainder to the states to make their own decisions how best to slash their programs.[84] Meanwhile, the AIDS epidemic, largely ignored by the White House, spread across the land. As reductions in federal funding decimated many public health programs, leaving Medicaid dollars to dominate the field, local health agencies spent much time and energy providing basic health services for the poor.

Twelve years after the Milbank Commission Report, the Institute of Medicine issued its own landmark report, *The Future of Public Health*.[85] This documented the bleak landscape of many public health departments across the country. Half of the state boards of health had disappeared; important programs had been taken away from health departments; and public health was "in disarray." The prose of this report was often vivid: "The most frequent perception of the health department by legislators and citizens was of a slow and inflexible bureaucracy battling with chaos, fighting to meet crises, and behaving in an essentially reactive manner. . . . Just getting through the day is the only real objective of the senior administrator."[86]

---

[82] *Ibid.*, p. 156.

[83] *Ibid.*, p. 212.

[84] G.S. Omenn, "What's Behind Those Block Grants in Health?" *New England Journal of Medicine*, 306, 1982, 1057–1060.

[85] Institute of Medicine, Committee for the Study of the Future of Public Health, *The Future of Public Health*. Washington, DC: National Academy Press, 1988, p. 6.

[86] *Ibid.*, p. 85.

The focus of the IOM report was on public health practice but it did have a number of recommendations for schools of public health, urging them to offer educational programs more targeted to the needs of practitioners. Schools of public health should establish firm practice links with state and local health departments so that more faculty members could undertake professional responsibilities in those agencies, conduct relevant research, and train students in practice situations. Just as had the Milbank report, so too the Institute of Medicine report urged schools of public health to serve as resources to government at all levels in the development of public health policy, to assist other types of institutions in educating public health practitioners, and to take better advantage of such university resources as schools of business administration and departments of physical, biological, and social sciences. Unlike the Milbank report, the Institute of Medicine committee asked schools of public health to provide short training courses and continuing education opportunities for public health practitioners. They also suggested that schools offer undergraduate courses in public health to attract recruits into the field. In summary, the task, as they defined it, was "to assist the schools in developing a greater emphasis on public health practice and to equip them to train personnel with the breadth of knowledge that matches the scope of public health."[87] The report especially highlighted the need for short courses to upgrade the skills of "that substantial majority of public health professionals who have not received appropriate formal training" and to ensure that all public health practitioners became aware of new knowledge and techniques. Nothing was said about designing a single rationally organized system of public health education.

In the years since the Institute of Medicine's report, the public health educational system has continued to expand at an accelerated pace. There are currently 31 accredited schools of public health and 45 accredited community health programs.[88] The Council on Education for Public Health estimates that the total number of accredited schools and programs may well double within the next ten years. The most dramatic growth is occurring outside the established schools of public health. Close to 40 percent of the nation's accredited medical schools now have operational M.P.H. programs or are currently developing a graduate public health degree program. New specializations are emerging such as human genetics, management of clinical trials, and public health informatics. Many schools and competing organizations are involved in distance learn-

---

[87] *Ibid.*, p. 157.

[88] This and the following details are derived from a presentation by Patricia P. Evans, "An Accreditation Perspective on the Future of Professional Public Health Preparation," to the Institute of Medicine Committee on Educating Public Health Professionals for the 21st Century, March 13, 2002, Irvine, California.

ing programs that offer the possibility of fulfilling the long-recognized need to bring public health education to the homes and offices of the public health workforce. The Internet also offers the possibility of bringing public health education to populations across the country and around the world; indeed, health information sites are among the most popular and frequently visited of all Web applications.

Is this a system badly in need of rational reconstruction or is it simply a system of dynamic, if sometimes messy, innovation—an academic marketplace evolving rapidly to meet the country's needs? Although it is not within the purview of the historian to answer such a question, it may be important to note one significant fact. Previous efforts to design truly effective systems of public health education generally foundered because of lack of political will, public disinterest, or paucity of funds. Since September 11, 2001, however, the context has changed dramatically. With public health riding high on the national agenda and an abundance of funds being promised, perhaps there is now an opportunity, as there has not been for a very long time, to shape a future system of public health education that addresses the problems that have been so often described and analyzed.

04/15/02

Appendix E

Occupational Classifications

Occupation	Federal Agencies	Voluntary Agencies	State and Territorial Agencies	Total
Administrators				
Health Administrator	1,152	—	14,768	15,920
Professionals				
Administrative/Business Professional	3,133	—	1,592	4,725
Attorney/Hearing Officer	351	—	250	601
Biostatistician	684	—	480	1,164
Clinical, Counseling, and School Psychologist	1	—	1	2
Environmental Engineer	3,092	—	1,457	4,549
Environmental Scientist & Specialist	3,951	—	10,931	14,882
Epidemiologist	5	—	922	927
Health Economist	86	—	19	105
Health Planner/Researcher/Analyst	2,074	—	1,499	3,573
Infection Control/Disease Investigator	2	—	781	783
Licensure/Inspection/Regulatory Specialist	9,625	—	4,155	13,780
Marriage and Family Therapist	—	—	—	—
Medical & Public Health Social Worker	170	—	2,006	2,176
Mental Health/Substance Abuse Social Worker	—	—	—	—

Occupation	Federal Agencies	Voluntary Agencies	State and Territorial Agencies	Total
Mental Health Counselor	113	—	673	786
Occupation Safety & Health Specialist	3,619	—	1,974	5,593
PH Dental Worker	1,240	—	792	2,032
PH Educator	126	—	2,104	2,230
PH Laboratory Professional	9,603	—	4,485	14,088
PH Nurse	4,311	8,000	36,921	49,232
PH Nutritionist	269	—	6,411	6,680
PH Optometrist	5	—	4	9
PH Pharmacist	1,180	—	316	1,496
PH Physical Therapist	12	—	60	72
PH Physician	4,055	—	1,953	6,008
PH Program Specialist	3,836	—	3,984	7,820
PH Student	37	—	14,996	15,033
PH Veterinarian/Animal Control Specialist	1,929	—	108	2,037
Psychiatric Nurse	—	—	4	4
Psychiatrist	—	—	1	1
Psychologist	688	—	67	755
Public Relations/Media Specialist	448	12	115	575
Substance Abuse & Behavioral Disorders Counselor	2	—	36	38
Other Public Health Professional	4,250	—	9,788	14,038
PH Professional, Title Unspecified	—	—	24,231	24,231
Technicians				
Computer Specialist	2,565	—	1,761	4,326
Environmental Engineering Technician	294	—	120	414
Environmental Science and Protection Technician	228	—	273	501
Health Information Systems/Data Analyst	172	—	433	605
Occupational Health and Safety Technician	93	—	2	95
PH Laboratory Specialist	4,262	—	1,438	5,700
Other Public Health Technician	4,081	—	22,872	26,953
Technician, Title Unspecified	—	—	2,916	2,916
Protective Service				
Investigations Specialist	326	—	50	376
Other or Unspecified Protective Service Worker	103	—	791	894

Occupation	Federal Agencies	Voluntary Agencies	State and Territorial Agencies	Total
Paraprofessionals				
Community Outreach/ Field Worker	102	—	574	676
Other or Unspecified Paraprofessional	1,134	—	17,768	18,902
Administrative Support				
Administrative Business Staff	2,498	—	1,285	3,783
Administrative Support Staff	9,343	—	28,462	37,805
Unspecified Clerical/ Support	—	—	10,324	10,324
Skilled Craft Workers				
Skilled Craft Worker	17	—	1,166	1,183
Service/Maintenance				
Food Services/House- Keeping	12	—	313	325
Patient Services	—	—	—	—
Other or Unspecified Service/Maintenance	32	—	4,363	4,395
Category Unreported				
Programs	—	7,202	7,052	14,254
Unidentifiable	443	171	97,268	97,882
Volunteers	—	2,864,825	5	2,864,830
Total w/Volunteers	85,754	2,880,210	347,120	3,313,084
Total w/o Volunteers	**85,754**	**15,385**	**347,115**	**448,254**

Appendix F

A Collection of Competency Sets

COMPETENCIES FOR PUBLIC HEALTH WORKERS:
A COLLECTION OF COMPETENCY SETS OF PUBLIC HEALTH-RELATED OCCUPATIONS AND PROFESSIONS

This table of competency sets of public health-related occupations and professions was produced by the Office of Workforce Policy and Planning (OWPP), Centers for Disease Control and Prevention (CDC) (www.phppo.cdc.gov/workforce) for the *Competencies and Curriculum Workgroup* of the *Public Health Workforce Development Progress Workshop* (June 18–19, 2001) and revised for the *Public Health Workforce Development Annual Meeting* (September 12–13, 2001).

This expansive table of known competency sets is intended to be a resource document for persons interested in public health workforce development and includes on-line sources for all documents listed. The competency sets listed can be used as an aid to curricula developers and instructional designers in planning training programs for the Nation's public health workers. These sets provide relevant examples of competency statements from occupations and professions that share in the work of public health. Used as a starting point, this list may help avoid duplication of efforts and build on the existing efforts among the many public health training centers across the U.S.

The competency sets are differentiated into the following categories:

- Core—Basic Public Health (addresses the essential services of public health)
- New Topical Areas (emergency response, genomics, law)
- Functional Areas (leadership, management, supervisory, secretarial)
- Discipline Specific (professional, technical, entry-level, student)
- Other Topical Areas (MCH, STD, etc.).

The competencies listed are those known at the time of printing. The comprehensive search for related public health worker competencies included numerous global and site-specific web searches, list-serv queries, and personal contacts. Since the field of workforce development is evolving, many competency sets—be they produced by government, academic institutions, public health and professional organizations—are in development. Therefore, this list may not contain all available competency sets. Inclusion of any competency set in the table does not imply Office of Workforce Policy and Planning endorsement.

Please notify Kimberly Geissman, KGeissman@cdc.gov, OWPP/CDC of major omissions, corrections, and additions.

A Collection of Competency Sets of Public Health-Related Occupations and Professions

Updated for the Public Health Workforce Development Annual Meeting, September 12–13, 2001, Athens, GA

Known Competency Sets	Worker Level[1]	Status and Where to Find Them
Core—Basic Public Health		
Competencies for Providing Essential Public Health Services, 1997	professional	The Public Health Workforce: An Agenda for the 21st Century, Public Health Functions Project, ODPHP,DHHS http://www.health.gov/phfunctions/publhlth.pdf essential services www.apha.org/ppp/science/10ES.htm
Council on Linkages: Core Competencies for Public Health Professionals 2001	front-line, senior professional, supervisor, manager	Public Health Foundation (PHF), http://www.trainingfinder.org/competencies/list.htm
Competencies for Providing Public Health Services, 1998	medical student	C.W. Keck, "Core Competencies for the Synergistic Practice of Medicine & Public Health" Josiah Macy, Jr., Foundation Conference, 1998 http://www.josiahmacyfoundation.org/jmacy1.html
Principles of Public Health course, 2001	leader, professional, technical	Based on Healthy People 2010, Missouri Public Health Training Network http://www.health.state.mo.us/series/
Public Health 101 course, 2000	professional	Based on Bernard Turnock's text Public Health: What It Is and How It Works, 2000. Illinois Center for Public Health Preparedness http://www.aspenpublishers.com/books/turnock/overview.html
Core competencies for MPH Students, 1998	MPH student	Johns Hopkins School of Public Health, Master of Public Health http://distance.jhsph.edu/mph/why/core_competencies.html
Masters of Public Health (MPH) in Health Behavior & Health Education	MPH student	University of Michigan School of Public Health, Department of Health Behavior and Health Education http://www.sph.umich.edu/hbhe/programs/mph.html
Document in development, 2001	MPH student	Deans of the Schools of Public Health, universal SPH competencies being drafted, contact Liz Weist http://www.asph.org/aa_document.cfm/5/5/172
New Topical Areas		
Emergency Response		
Core Public Health Worker Competencies for Emergency Preparedness and Response, April 2001	leader, administrator, professional, technical, support	Center for Health Policy, Columbia University School of Nursing http://cpmcnet.columbia.edu/dept/nursing/institute-centers/chphsr/COMPETENCIES.pdf

Fire & Emergency Services Competency Module	technical	Industry-Specific Competency Modules, KnowledgePoint http://www.knowledgepoint.com/products/firecomp.html
Genomics		
Genomics Competencies for the Public Health Workforce, May 2001	administrator, professional,* all workers (technical, support)	Office of Genetics and Disease Prevention and Public Health Practice Program Office, CDC http://www.cdc.gov/genetics/training/competencies/ *(clinicians, educators, environmental workers, epidemiologists, laboratorians),
Competencies in Public Health Genetics, June 1999	MPH, MS, PhD student	"Public Health Genetics In the Content of Law, Ethics and Policy" Program, Institute for Public Health Genetics, Public Health Genetics Training Collaboration (CDC, HRSA funded) http://depts.washington.edu/phgen/DegreeTracks/competencies.html
Core Competencies in Genetics Essential for All Health Care Professionals, February 2000	all health care professional, student	National Coalition for Health Professional Education in Genetics (NCHPEG), (RWJ, DOE funded) http://www.nchpeg.org/news-box/corecompetencies000.html
Medical School Core Curriculum in Genetics, 1995	medical student	American Society of Human Genetics (ASHG) http://www.ashg.org/genetics/ashg/policy/rep-01.htm
Law		
Core Legal Competencies for Public Health Practitioners, June 2001	health official, governance boards, front-line, senior-level professional, supervisor, manager	Center for Law and Public's Health at Johns Hopkins and Georgetown Universities (with CDC, PHF) http://www.publichealthlaw.net/Training/Methods.htm
Functional Areas		
Leadership		
Public Health Leadership Competency Framework, August 2000	health director, health officer	Public Health Leadership Network (PHLN), CDC http://www.slu.edu/organizations/nln/competency_framework.html Wright, K. Rowitz, L., Merkle, A., et al. "Competency Development in Public Health", *American Journal of Public Health*, August 2000, vol 90, no 8.

Project Management Body of Knowledge (PMBOK Guide), 2000	leader, project manager	Public Health Leadership Institute (PHLI), CDC http://www.phls.org Guide found at Project Management Institute http://www.pmi.org/publictn/pmboktoc.htm
Leadership Competencies for Assistant Deputy Ministers and Senior Executives	senior manager	The Learning Centre, Public Service Commission of Canada http://www.psc-cfp.gc.ca/aexdp/leaders_e.htm
Leadership Development Competencies: The Leadership Challenge	leader	Exploring Inspired Leadership, The Banff Center http://www.banffmanagement.com
Management		
Core Competencies for Supervisors, Managers, and Executives, 2000	director, executive, team leader, program manager, supervisor	School of Public Health Leadership & Management Development, CDC Corporate University; Vicki Johnson, HRMO, VJohnson1@cdc.gov http://intranet.cdc.gov/hrmo/masdevpl.htm
Supervisors' and Managers' Critical Elements, October 1999	supervisor, manager	Headquarters Performance Management System, DOE http://www.hr.doe.gov/hqpms/supstan.htm
Management Academy for Public Health Competencies, March 1999	public & private sector manager	Management Academy for Public Health (MAPH), North Carolina Institute for Public Health (CDC, HRSA, Kellogg, RWJ funded); http://www.maph.unc.edu Stephen Orton sorton@email.unc.edu
Competency Profile: Public Service Managers	middle-managers	The Learning Centre, Profile for Leaders and Managers, Public Service Commission, Canada http://learnet.gc.ca/eng/comcentr/manage/profile/auto.htm
Public Health Prevention Service Competency Set, September 1997	MS-prepared entry-level manager	Public Health Prevention Service (PHPS) Fellowship, CDC (to be updated fall 2001) http://www.cdc.gov/epo/dapht/rfa.htm#perform
Competencies for Professional Development: Managing in the Middle, 1998	mid-level manager	Exploring Inspired Leadership, The Banff Center http://www.banffmanagement.com
Secretary – Support		
Competencies for Secretary and Office Automation Clerk (GS-318, GS-326), 2000	secretary, office automation clerk	School of Public Health Business Management, CDC Corporate University; Jessi Stevens, HRMO JStevens@cdc.gov http://intranet.cdc.gov/hrmo/crses.htm
Sample Elements and Tasks for Secretary	secretary	Headquarters Performance Management System, DOE http://www.hr.doe.gov/hqpms.secy.htm

National Competency Standards – Public Administration, Competency Based Assessment and Training Handbook, 1999	mid-level administrator, clerical	Office of the Commissioner for Public Employment, Australia's Northern Territory Government http://www.nt.gov.au/ocpe/documents/people-development/comp-standards
CASAS Competency List	basic life skills	Secretary's's Commission on Achieving Necessary Skills, DOL http://www.casas.org/01AboutCasas/01Competencies.html
High School Student Competencies and Indicators	high school graduate	National Occupational Information Coordinating Committee (NOICC), Academic Innovations http://www.academicinnovations.com/noicc.html

Discipline Specific

Epidemiology

Health Science and Epidemiology Competencies, 2001	professional	School of Public Health Science and Research, CDC Corporate University, draft to be validated; Charlotte Wilson, HRMO CWilson@cdc.gov
Core Activities for Learning (CALS)	doctoral-level Epidemic Intelligence Officer	Epidemic Intelligence Service (EIS), CDC Jim Alexander, EPO/DAPHT JAlexander1@cdc.gov
Evaluation of EIS Competency Domains: Epidemiologic Process, Communication, and Professionalism, 2001	doctoral-level Epidemic Intelligence Officer	Epidemic Intelligence Service (EIS), CDC Jim Alexander, EPO/DAPHT JAlexander1@cdc.gov
Maternal and Child Health Epidemiology Fellowship Competency Guidelines	professional	Council of State and Territorial Epidemiologists (CSTE) with CDC http://www.cste.org/MCHcompetencies.pdf
Infection Control and Epidemiology: Professional and Practice Standards, 1998	professional	Association for Practitioners in Infection Control & Epidemiology (APIC) and Community and Hospital Infection Control Association, Canada (CHICA) http://www.apic.org/pdf/pracstnd.pdf

Informatics

Public Health Informatics Competencies, 2001	professional	CDC, draft in development; Patrick O'Carroll, PHPPO POCarroll@cdc.gov
Information Resources Management Competencies, 2001	professional, technical	School of Public Health Information Resources Management, CDC Corporate University, draft to be validated; Tonya Henderson, HRMO TSHenderson@cdc.gov

Competency	Audience	Source
Math and Statistical Competencies, 2001	professional, technical	School of Public Health Science & Research, CDC Corporate University, draft to be validated; Charlotte Wilson, HRMO CWilson@cdc.gov
Recommendations of the International Medical Informatics Association (IMIA) on Education in Health and Medical Informatics, October 2000	physician, nurse, pharmacist, manager, record administrator, teacher, student	American Medical Informatics Association (AMIA), Health and Medical Informatics Education Workgroup http://www.amia.org/ updated: introductory, intermediate, advanced levels, found at International Medical Informatics Association (IMIA) http://www.rzuser.uni-heidelberg.de/~d16/rec.htm
Registered Health Information Administrator (RHIA) and RHIT (technician) Examination Content: Domains, Subdomains and Tasks	administrator, technical	American Healthcare through Quality Information (AMIMA) http://www.ahima.org/certification/exam.html
Certified Coding Specialist (CCS) Coding Competencies	coder	American Healthcare through Quality Information (AMIMA) http://www.ahima.org/certification/exam.html
Medical School Objectives Project: Medical Informatics Objectives, August 2000	MD student	Association of American Medical Colleges (AAMC), School Objectives Project http://www.aamc.org/meded/msop/informat.htm
On-line Technology Competencies	undergraduate student	College of Education and Applied Professions, Western Carolina University http://www.ceap.wcu.edu/Martin/Compdef.htm
Student Technology Competency Matrix	high school graduate	Millbury Public Schools http://millbury.k12.ma.us/~hs/school/techplan/studentmatrix4.3B.html

Environment

Competency	Audience	Source
Environmental Health Competency Project: Recommendations for Core Competencies for Local Environmental Health Practitioners, May 2001	front-line, local-level professional	American Public Health Association (APHA) and National Center for Environmental Health (NCEH/CDC) with NEHA, NACCHO, ASTHO, FCA, AAS, NALBOH, final draft in clearance June 1, report due August 2001. Patrick Bohan, NCEH PBohan@cdc.gov http://www.apha.org/ppp/ehproject.htm
Environmental Health Competencies: Core Competencies for the Effective Practice of Environmental Health	professional	Funding Opportunity, Association of School of Public Health (ASPH), Developing Communities of Excellence in Environmental Health http://www.asph.org/fac_document.cfm/69/69/5968
Registered Environmental Health Specialist/Registered Sanitarian Examination	entry-level professional	National Environmental Health Association (NEHA), exam content outline; Ryan Rudolph rrudolph@neha.org http://www.neha.org

Engineering		
Sample Elements and Tasks for Engineer, October 1999	professional	Headquarters Performance Management System, DOE http://www.hr.doe.gov/hqpms/engineer.htm
Health Education		
Responsibilities & Competencies for Health Educators, 1997	professional	Nat'l Commission for Health Education Credentialing (NCHEC), endorsed by Society for Public Health Education (SOPHE), American Association for Health Education (AAHE), Association of State and Territorial Directors of Health Promotion and Public Health Education (ASTDHPPHE) update due August 2001, http://www.nchec.org/competencies.htm
Core Competencies/ "The Extension Educator"	professional	Department of Agriculture and Natural Resources Education and Communication Systems (ANRECS), Michigan State University, staff professional development http://www.anrecs.msu.edu/extension/profdev/10areas.htm
Communications		
Public Health Education and Communication Competencies, August 2000	manager, public relations specialist, visual information specialist, technical writer, editor, audio-video technician	School of Public Health Education and Communication, CDC Corporate University; Christopher Stallard HRMO http://intranet.cdc.gov/hrmo/masdev2.htm
Library and Information Science		
Information Literacy Competency Standards for Higher Education, January 2000	undergraduate student	Association of College and Research Libraries (ACRL), American Library Association (ALA), http://www.ala.org/acrl/ilcomstan.html
Competencies for Special Librarians of the 21st Century, 1998	entry-level professional	Special Libraries Association (SLA), supported by Association for Library and Information Science Education (ALISE) and Medical Library Association (MLA) http://www.sla.org/content/memberservice/researchforum/lisprograms/lisps.cfm

273

Title	Role	Source
Students' Information Literacy Needs in the 21st Century: Competencies for Teacher-Librarians	teacher-librarian, high school student	Association for Teacher-Librarianship in Canada (ATLC) http://www.atlc.ca/Publications/competen.htm
Knowledge and Skills for Entry-Level	entry-level technical	American Library Association (ALA), Association for Library Collections & Technical Service (ALCTS), Committee on Education, Training and Recruitment for Cataloging http://www.uky.edu/~lhjeng00/cetrccmp.htm
Human Resources		
Human Resource Competencies for the Year 2000: A Professionals' Toolkit for Professional Development	professional	Northeast Human Resources Association, (NEHRA), www.nehra.com/about.php3 Society for Human Resource Management (SHRM) book, profiles of 31 competencies http://shrm.org/competencies/home.htm
Human Resources Management Competencies, 2001	leader, manager, professional	School of Public Health Business Management, CDC Corporate University, draft to be validated; Jessi Stevens, HRMO JStevens@cdc.gov
Directory of Competencies for the Human Resources Community in the Public Service of Canada, October 1998	professional	The Learning Centre, Public Service Commission, Canada http://learnet.gc.ca/eng/lrncentr/index.htm
Human Resource Competency Model	manager	International Personnel Management Association (IPMA), 22 competencies http://ipma-hr.org/public/training_template.cfm?ID=12
Laboratory		
Body of Knowledge	laboratorian, specialist, phlebotomist, technician	American Society of Clinical Laboratory Science (ASCLS), book, competencies for CLS and CLT regardless of setting, http://www.ascls.org/index.htm
Nutrition – Dietetics		
Core Competencies for the Supervised Practice Component of Entry-Level Dietician (Technician) Programs, 1997	dietitian student, dietetic technician student	Commission on Accreditation for Dietetics Education, "Accreditation Manual for Dietetics Education Programs, Revised 4th Edition," Catalog #6107 http://www.eatright.org/cade/standards.html
Standards of Professional Practice for Dietetics Professionals	dietitian	American Dietetics Association (ADA) http://www.eatright.org/qm/standardslist.html

Physical Activity

Athletic Training Clinical Proficiencies, 1999	entry-level professional, student	National Athletic Trainer's Association (NATA) http://www.nata.org, clinical focus
Physical Education for Lifelong Fitness, course	teacher, director, student	"Athletic Training Educational Competencies" http://www.cewl.com/ American Alliance for Health, Physical Education, Recreation & Dance (AAHPERD) http://www.aahperd.org curriculum book http://americanfitness.net/Physical_Best/
Standards of Competence, August 2000	therapist	Federation of State Boards of Physical Therapy http://www.fsbpt.org/news.htm

Medicine

Preventive Medicine Residency (PMR) Competency Matrix, 2000–2001	MD-trained, Preventive Medicine Resident	Preventive Medicine Residency Program (PMR), CDC Jim Lando, EPO/DAPHT JLando@cdc.gov
Core Competencies and Performance Indicators for Preventive Medicine Residents, 1999	MD-trained, Preventive Medicine Resident	American College of Preventive Medicine (ACPM) with HRSA http://www.acpm.org/corecomp.htm
Occupational and Environmental Medicine Competencies, January 1998	physician administrator, generalist, specialist	American College of Occupational and Environmental Medicine (ACOEM) http://www.acoem.org/paprguid/guides/comp.htm
An Inventory of Knowledge and Skills Relating to Disease Prevention and Health Promotion, 1989	MD student	Association of Teachers of Preventive Medicine (ATPM) http://www.atpm.org/library/inventory/inventory1.htm
Competencies at the Terre Haute Center for Medical Education: Competency Definitions	MA-MD student	Terre Haute Center for Medical Education, Indiana University School of Medicine http://web.indstate.edu/thcme/duong/Competency/Definitions.html

Nursing

Public Health Nursing Practice for the 21st Century, 2001	professional	Minnesota Department of Health, Division of Nursing and University of Minnesota, School of Nursing (HRSA-funded) draft tool for assessment, undergoing validation by the Association of State and Territorial Directors of Nursing (ASTDN) and Association of Community Health Nurse Educator (ACHNE); Derryl Block dblock@d.umn.edu

Title	Level	Source
National Competency Standards for the Registered Nurse, 2000	registered nurse, student	Australian Nursing Council, Inc. (ANCI) http://www.anci.org.au/competencystandards.htm
Delivery of Occupational and Environmental Health Services, May 1998	nurse professional	American Association of Occupational Health Nursing (AAOHN) http://www.aaohn.org/servicedelivery_position.htm
Dentistry *Competency Statements for Dental Public Health, September 1997*	professional	American Association of Public Health Dentistry (AAPHD) http://www.pitt.edu/~aaphd/dph.competency.html
Pharmacy *Certification in Geriatric Pharmacy Practice: Content Guide, 1997*	professional	"Certified Geriatric Pharmacist: A Bridge to Enhanced Respect, Expanded Responsibility— and More" by David K. Buerger http://www.ascp.com/public/pubs/tcp/1997/jun/gerpharm.html
Competency Statements: Disease State Management (DSM) Examinations	professional	National Association of Boards of Pharmacy (NABP) http://www.nabp.net/
Behavioral/Social Science *Behavioral & Social Science Competencies,* draft 2001	professional	School of Public Health Science and Research, CDC Corporate University, draft to be validated; Charlotte Wilson, HRMO CWilson@cdc.gov
Description of the Doctoral Program: Educational Objectives	PhD students	School of Social Work, University of North Carolina at Chapel Hill, learning objectives http://www.sowo.unc.edu/doctoral/description/index.html
Ethical Principles of Psychologists and Code of Conduct, December 1992	professional	American Psychological Association (APA), "General Principles" http://www.apa.org/ethics/code.html
Biological Science *Biological Science Competencies,* draft 2001	professional	School of Public Health Science and Research, CDC Corporate University, draft to be validated; Charlotte Wilson, HRMO CWilson@cdc.gov
Public Health Advisor Series *Competencies for Public Health Advisors (GS-685), 2001*	professional	School of Public Health Administration, CDC Corporate University, intranet assessment of 1) foundation competencies and 2) occupational competencies; Ronald Lake, HRMO RLake@cdc.gov

Program Analysis/Evaluation

Competencies for Public Health Analyst (GS-685), 2001	professional	School of Public Health Administration, CDC Corporate University, draft to be validated; Ronald Lake, HRMO RLake@cdc.gov http://intranet.cdc.gov/hrmo/analyst.htm
Career Development: Core Competencies (Evaluation and Inspections), December 1999	manager, program analyst, team leader, administrator, technical support, secretary	Office of Evaluation and Inspections (OEI), Office of Inspector General (OIG), http://www.hhs.gov/oig/oei/evaluator/evaluator.html

Policy Analysis

Generic Policy Analyst Draft Competency Profile	professional	The Learning Centre, Public Service Commission, Canada http://learnet.gc.ca/eng/lrncentr/index.htm

Economics

Nebraska Standards in Business Education Essential Leanings: Focus on Economics	student, public	EcEd Economics Education Web competencies and learning objectives http://ecedweb.unomaha.edu/standards/home.htm
National and State Content Standards in Economics	student, public	EconomicsAmerica, National Council on Economic Education (NCEE), 20 standards, learning objectives and performance benchmarks http://www.economicsamerica.org

Finance

Core Competency Framework for Entry into the Accounting Profession: Functional Competencies	entry-level professional	American Institute of Certified Public Accountants (AICPA) http://www.aicpa.org/edu/func.htm
Competency Model for the New Finance Professional	professional, technical, support	American Institute of Certified Public Accountants (AICPA) tool being piloted http://www.cpatoolbox.org
Core Competencies (future of the CPA profession), 2001	professional, technical	Vision Project Team and State Societies, CPA Vision Project: 2001 and Beyond http://www.cpavision.org

Other Topical Areas

	Category	Source
Community-based Health		
Community Health Scholars Program: Goal and Competencies, June 1999	post-doctoral student	Community-Based Public Health (CBPH), University of Michigan School of Public Health, Kellogg sponsored, program competencies http://www.sph.umich.edu/chsp/goal.html
MCH		
Maternal and Child Health Competencies, February 2001	professional	Association of Teachers of Maternal and Child Health (ATMCH) http://www.atmch.org/mchcomps.pdf
Cultural/Diversity		
The Provision of Culturally Competent Health Care	leader, professional, technical, support	Amy V. Blue, PhD., Assistant Dean for Curriculum and Evaluation, Medical University of South Carolina College of Medicine http://www.musc.edu/deansclerkship/rccultur.html
Bridge to Wellness: Cultural Competency	clinician	Evelyn Lee, EdD, Executive Director of Richmond Area Multi-Services, Inc. (RAMS) http://www.serve.com/Wellness/culture.html
STD/HIV		
Program Operations Guidelines for STD Prevention: Training and Professional Developments	clinician, disease investigator, HIV counseling	Center for HIV, STD, and TB Prevention, CDC; Frankie Barnes, NCHSTP/DSTD FBarnes@cdc.gov http://www.cdc.gov/std/program/training.pdf

[1]Categories: Leader, Professional, Technical, Support. *The Public Health Work Force Enumeration 2000,* National Center for Health Workforce Information and Analysis, HRSA, DHHS. (Order document at http://www.ask.hrsa.gov/detail.cfm?id=BHP00079, download at http://cpmcnet.columbia.edu/dept/nursing/chphsr/enum2000.pdf.)

Appendix G

Public Meetings

**COMMITTEE ON EDUCATING PUBLIC HEALTH PROFESSIONALS
FOR THE 21ST CENTURY
MEETING I
NOVEMBER 14, 2001**

Agenda

8:30 am – 9:30 am Discussion of Committee Charge
Presentation of Charge by RWJ
J. Michael McGinnis, M.D., Senior Vice
President and Director, Health Group
Pamela Williams Russo, M.D., M.P.H.

COMMITTEE ON EDUCATING PUBLIC HEALTH PROFESSIONALS FOR THE 21ST CENTURY MEETING II JANUARY 23, 2002

Agenda

1:00 pm	Workforce Development: Issues and Approaches CDC efforts on public health workforce development Maureen Lichtveld, M.D., M.P.H.
1:30 pm	HRSA efforts in public health education and training Sam Shekar, M.D., M.P.H.
2:00 pm	The professional workforce—where do they work and what do they need to know? Virginia Kennedy, Ph.D.
2:30 pm	Discussion
3:00 pm	Break
3:15 pm	*Panel on Issues and Questions from the Field*—Each presenter has 15–20 minutes to describe his/her perspective on what schools of public health need to do to prepare public health professionals to meet the challenges of public health in the 21st century. Discussion will follow completion of all presentations. American Public Health Association (APHA)— Mohammad Akhter, M.D., M.P.H. Public Health Foundation (PHF)—Ronald Bialek, M.P.P. Society of Public Health Education (SOPHE)—Elaine Auld, M.P.H. Public Health DrPH Programs—Vaughn Upshaw, Ed.D., Dr.P.H., UNC, School of Public Health
4:30 pm	Discussion
5:00 pm	At this time any others who may be in attendance will be provided the opportunity to ask questions and participate in the discussion.
5:30 pm	Adjourn

Speakers

Mohammad Akhter, M.D., M.P.H.
Executive Director
American Public Health Association (APHA)

Elaine Auld, M.P.H.
Executive Director
Society of Public Health Education (SOPHE)

Ronald Bialek, M.P.P.
Executive Director
Public Health Foundation (PHF)

Virginia Kennedy, Ph.D.
Associate Professor, Management & Policy Sciences
Associate Director, Center for Health Policy Studies
University of Texas, Houston School of Public Health

Maureen Lichtveld, M.D., M.P.H.
Associate Director for Workforce Development
Centers for Disease Control (CDC)

Sam Shekar, M.D., M.P.H.
Associate Administrator, Bureau of Health Professions
Health Resources and Services Administration (HRSA)

Vaughn Upshaw, Ed.D., Dr.P.H.
Director, Public Health DrPH Programs
University of North Carolina School of Public Health

COMMITTEE ON EDUCATING PUBLIC HEALTH PROFESSIONALS FOR THE 21ST CENTURY
MEETING III
MARCH 13–14, 2002

Agenda

March 13, 2002

8:00 am   Welcome and Introductions of Guests

8:15 am – 9:30 pm Presentations and Discussion—Views on what
                          M.P.H. programs and what schools of public health
                          need to do to prepare public health professionals to
                          meet the challenges of public health in the 21st
                          century.
                          Harrison Spencer, M.D., M.P.H., Association of
                             Schools of Public Health
                          Patricia P. Evans, M.P.H., Executive Director,
                             Council on Education for Public Health

March 14, 2002

8:00 am – 8:45 pm Ethics and Public Health
                          James Thomas, Ph.D., UNC School of Public Health

Speakers

Patricia P. Evans, M.P.H.
Executive Director
Council on Education for Public Health (CEPH)

Harrison Spencer, M.D., M.P.H.
Executive Director
Association of Schools of Public Health (ASPH)

James Thomas, Ph.D.
Associate Professor of Epidemiology
Director of the Program in Public Health Ethics
University of North Carolina School of Public Health

COMMITTEE ON EDUCATING PUBLIC HEALTH PROFESSIONALS
FOR THE 21ST CENTURY
MEETING IV
MAY 23, 2002

Agenda

8:30 am   Public Health Education in Accredited Programs
                       William Livingood, Ph.D.
                       State Department of Health Florida

8:50 am – 9:15 am Discussion

Appendix H

Committee Biographies

Kristine Gebbie, DrPH, RN (co-chair) is Director of the Center for Health Policy and the Doctor of Nursing Science Program, as well as Elizabeth Standish Gill Associate Professor of Nursing at Columbia University. She has conducted extensive research on health policy, public health nurses, and public health laws, and is a recognized expert in the enumeration and development of the public health workforce. Dr. Gebbie is an IOM member with expertise in public health systems and infrastructures, HIV/AIDS prevention policy development, state and local public health practice, and public health nursing. She was elected to the IOM in 1992.

Linda Rosenstock, MD, MPH (co chair) is currently Dean of the UCLA School of Public Health. She holds academic appointments as professor of medicine in the School of Medicine and professor of environmental health sciences in the School of Public Health. She served as Director of the National Institute for Occupational Safety and Health (NIOSH) (1994–2000) and in 2000, Dr. Rosenstock received the Presidential Distinguished Executive Award. She has been active in clinical primary care, internal medicine, and occupational medicine, and also is active internationally in teaching and research in occupational and environmental health, serving as an advisor to the World Health Organization. She was elected to the IOM in 1995.

Susan M. Allan, JD, MD, MPH is the Health Director for the Department of Human Services in Arlington County, Virginia. Dr. Allan has extensive experience in planning, development, organization, and direction of public health initiatives. Prior to her promotion to Arlington County Health Director, Dr. Allan was the county's Medical Supervisor of Public Health Clinics, and the Public Health Physician. She was a scholar in the inaugural year of the Centers for Disease Control's Public Health Leadership Institute. She has also had medical training in small rural clinics in such developing countries as Colombia. Dr. Allan has presented widely and published in health issues related to immigrants and refugees, local and state roles in public health care services, and leadership and health care. She has been very active in a number of capacities with the National Association of County and City Health Officials and is also the NACCHO representative to the Council on Linkages between Academia and Public Health Practice. Most recently, she served on the Committee on Leading Health Indicators for *Healthy People 2010.*

Kaye Bender, PhD, RN was appointed Deputy State Health Officer for the Mississippi State Department of Health in October 1998. As Deputy, Dr. Bender is second in command of the statewide public health system. Previous to this position, Dr. Bender served 10 years as the Chief of Staff of the State Health Officer at the Mississippi State Department of Health. Her responsibilities included directing the offices of Policy and Planning, Public Health Nursing, Field Services, Primary Care Development, among others. Over her professional career, Dr. Bender has served in leadership positions as Director of Public Health Nursing, Field Services Nurse Consultant, District V Supervising Nurse, and Maternal-Child Health Nurse Consultant with the Mississippi State Department of Health. Dr. Bender is active in the American Nurses Association, Mississippi Nurses Association, American Public Health Association, and the Association of State and Territorial Health Officials Senior Deputies.

Dan G. Blazer, III, MD, PhD, MPH is JP Gibbons professor of Psychiatry and Behavioral Sciences at Duke University Medical Center. During Dr. Blazer's tenure as Dean of Medical Education at Duke, he expanded a Master of Public Health program for medical school students which now attracts over 20 percent of the medical school class. Dr. Blazer is the author or editor of over 25 books and author or co-author of over 260 peer-reviewed articles on topics including depression, epidemiology, and consultation liaison psychiatry. He is a fellow of the American College of Psychiatry and the American Psychiatric Association with expertise in geriatric psychiatry medical education, religion and medicine, preventive medicine, and public health. He was elected to the IOM in 1995.

Scott Burris, JD is on the faculty of the Temple University Beasley School of Law in Philadelphia, and is Associate Director of the Center for Law and the Public's Health at Georgetown and Johns Hopkins Universities. He was formerly an attorney at the American Civil Liberties Union of Pennsylvania and is a graduate of Yale Law School. He serves on numerous advisory committees on matters relating to public health law and has published extensively on the subject in both health and legal journals. He is the editor of *AIDS Law Today: A New Guide for the Public* (1993). His research has been supported by grants from funders including the Robert Wood Johnson Foundation, the Open Society Institute, the American Foundation for AIDS Research, and the CDC.

Mark Cullen, MD is Professor of Medicine and Public Health and Program Director of the Occupational and Environmental Medicine Program at Yale University School of Medicine. His two areas of research focus include occupational asthma and the relationship between socioeconomic status and health, with an emphasis on the role of work organization. Dr. Cullen serves as consultant to several large corporations, unions and non-profit organizations. At the IOM, he has been active on committees relating to manpower, training, and curricula in occupational and environmental medicine; and has been a peer reviewer on publications concerning Agent Orange and the Persian Gulf War. He serves on the IOM Health Sciences Policy Board. Dr. Cullen has published extensively in numerous journals and co-edited two textbooks. He received his MD from Yale. He was elected to the IOM in 1997.

Haile Tesfaye Debas, MD is Dean of the School of Medicine and Vice Chancellor for Medical Affairs at the University of California, San Francisco. He is an IOM member and currently serves on the Membership Committee. His expertise is in academic medicine and he has a keen interest in education. He is a gifted teacher who brought the Department of Surgery at UCSF to previously unprecedented national recognition, which is now considered one of the best academic departments of surgery in the country. The recipient of continuous NIH funding, Dean Debas has national recognition as a gastrointestinal investigator and has made numerous original contributions to medicine. Dr. Debas received his MD from McGill University School of Medicine. He was elected to the IOM in 1990.

Robert Goodman, PhD, MPH, MA holds an Endowed Professorship in the Department of Community Health Sciences at the Tulane University School of Public Health and Tropical Medicine. Formerly he was Director of the Center for Community Research at the Wake Forest University School of Medicine and a faculty member at the University of North

Carolina and the University of South Carolina Schools of Public Health. Dr. Goodman has written extensively on issues concerning community health development, community coalitions, evaluation methods, organizational development, and the institutionalization of health programs. He has been the principal investigator and evaluator on projects for the CDC, the National Cancer Institute, the Centers for Substance Abuse Prevention, the Office on Women's Health, the Children's Defense Fund, and several state health departments.

Alan Guttmacher, MD is the Deputy Director of the National Human Genome Research Institute (NHGRI) of the National Institutes of Health. In that role, he helps oversee the NHGRI's efforts in advancing genome research, integrating the benefits of genome research into health care, and exploring the ethical, legal, and social implications of human genomics. He also serves as Director of the NHGRI's Office of Policy, Planning, and Communications and thus directs the institute's health affairs, public policy, communications, and public education functions. Dr. Guttmacher formerly was at the University of Vermont, where his roles included directing the Vermont Regional Genetics Center, the Vermont Human Genetics Initiative, the Vermont Cancer Center's Familial Cancer Program, the Vermont Newborn Screening Program, and the NIH-supported Community Genetics and Ethics Initiative, the nation's first statewide effort to involve the general public in discussing the Human Genome Project's ethical, legal and social implications. A graduate of Harvard College and Harvard Medical School, Dr. Guttmacher completed a residency in Pediatrics and a fellowship in Medical Genetics at Children's Hospital of Boston and Harvard. He is a fellow of the American Academy of Pediatrics and of the American College of Medical Genetics.

Rita Kukafka, DrPH, MA is Assistant Professor, jointly appointed with the Mailman School of Pubic Health (Sociomedical Sciences) and the Department of Medical Informatics, College of Physicians and Surgeons at Columbia University. The focus of her dual appointment is to develop a program of research and training in Public Health Informatics. She holds a Doctorate degree from the School of Public Health at Columbia University and two masters degrees, one in health education, and the second in Medical Informatics from Columbia University, where she also completed a National Library of Medicine awarded postdoctoral fellowship in Medical Informatics. Her research focuses on representing patient perceptions and beliefs for purposes of creating patient-tailored information, computer mediated communications designed to influence changes in health behaviors and provider practices, and how theory from the behavioral sciences can be applied to advance our understanding and to improve our capacity to implement information technology systems into health care organizations.

Roxanne Parrott, PhD is a Professor in the Department of Communication Arts & Sciences and Director of the Health Communication Program at Pennsylvania State University. She is currently principal investigator of a CDC-funded grant that examines strategies for communicating genetics information to the lay public and co-investigator for an ELSI grant that examines the ethical and social implications of race-based pharmacogenomic messages. Her previous funded research focused on cancer communications, emphasizing social influence theories and community-based models in health message design and evaluation. She was the co-recipient of a Linkages Award in 1999 from NACCHO and ASTHO in recognition of an innovative national model of collaboration between public health agencies and institutions of higher learning. Dr. Parrott has published extensively, including the award-winning volume cited in the 2010 Chapter on Health Communication, "Designing Health Messages: Approaches from Communication Theory and Public Health Practice," and "Evaluating Women's Health Messages: A Resource Book."

Sheila M. Smythe, MS is Executive Vice President of New York Medical College and Dean of the School of Public Health, President of the Partnership for a Healthy Population, and Professor of Health Policy and Economics. Formerly, Ms. Smythe held the position of Chief Health Policy Advisor of the US General Accounting Office, was President and Chief Operating Officer of Empire Blue Cross and Blue Shield in New York, and Assistant Director of Research and Planning for the Blue Cross and Blue Shield Association.

William A. Vega, PhD is Director of the Behavioral and Research Training Institute of University Behavioral HealthCare of the Robert Wood Johnson Medical School. He is also a member of the faculty at the Robert Wood Johnson Medical School, University of Medicine & Dentistry of New Jersey. Formerly, Dr. Vega was Professor of Public Health at the University of California at Berkeley. He was recipient of the 2002 Community, Culture, and Prevention Science Award from the Society for Prevention Research, and the 2002 Award for Excellence in Research from the National Hispanic Science Network (sponsored by the National Institute of Drug Abuse). He received his academic degrees in sociology and criminology from the University of California at Berkeley. Dr. Vega's expertise is comparative studies of ethnicity and health, with a specialization in immigrant adaptation and behavioral health adjustments that occur among Latino adolescents and adults. He is currently interested in the paradox: "How do impoverished Hispanics achieve superior health profiles compared to native born Hispanics and European Americans?"

Patricia W. Wahl, PhD is Dean of the School of Public Health and Community Medicine at the University of Washington in Seattle where she is also Professor of Biostatistics. She previously served as Associate Dean of the School and as Acting Chair of the Department of Pathobiology. Currently, she is a member of the Administrative Committee of the Council on Education in Public Health (CEPH), the accrediting agency for schools of public health and graduate public health programs. In 1999 Dr. Wahl received the American Public Health Association's Statistics Section Award for outstanding contributions to the field of statistics and public health in administration, research, and training. Dr. Wahl is a member of the IOM Board on Health Promotion and Disease Prevention.

Index

G

H

AAO-8708